AMERICAN JOURNAL of PUBLIC HEALTH
MAY 2024
Issue 5

AJPH

A PUBLICATION OF THE
AMERICAN PUBLIC HEALTH ASSOCIATION

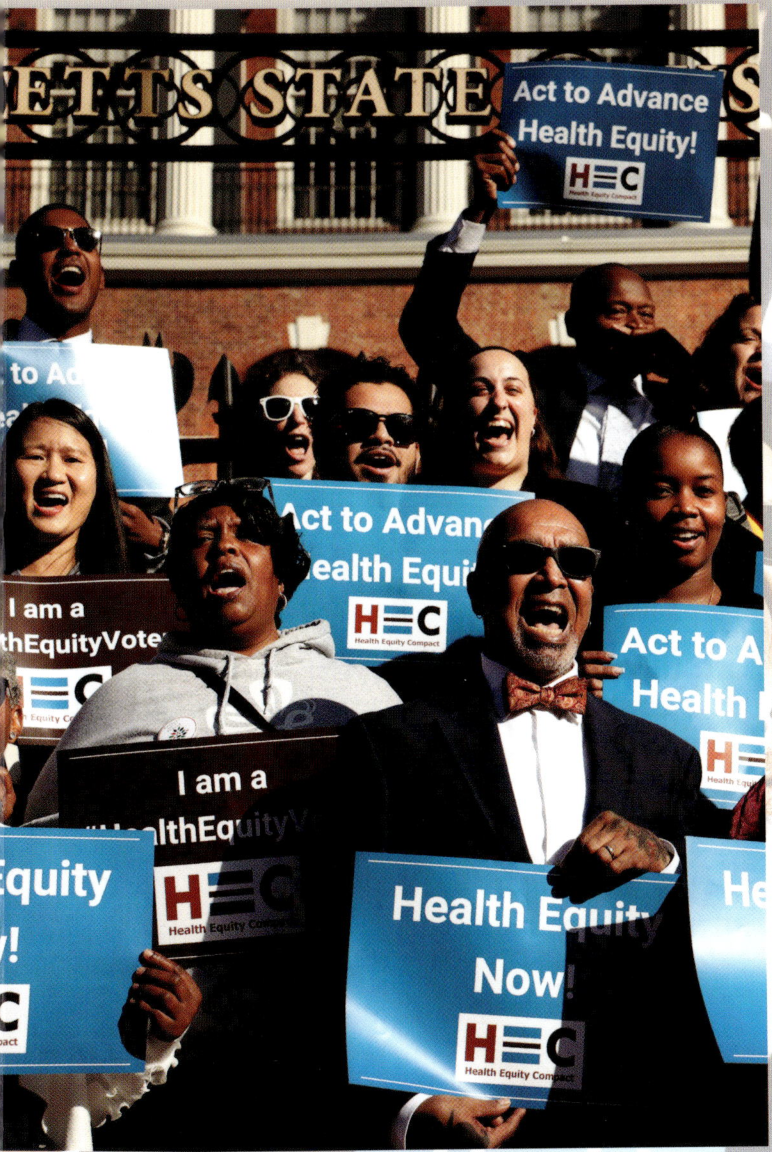

REVISITING THE 1988 FUTURE OF PUBLIC HEALTH: PROGRESS AND LIMITATIONS

The Good, the Bad, and the Ugly, pp. 453 and 479
Progress, pp. 467 and 495
Impact on CDC, p. 489
National Health Service, p. 471
Climate Change, p. 476
Studying vs Acting, p. 486

Also in this issue:

MENTAL HEALTH
Trajectories During COVID-19, p. 511
Trends by Gender Identity, p. 523

US CARCERAL SYSTEM
Per- and Polyfluoroalkyl Exposure, p. 501

APHA
AMERICAN PUBLIC HEALTH ASSOCIATION
For science. For action. For health.

AJPH®, published monthly, is the official Journal of the American Public Health Association®, 800 I St NW, Washington, DC 20001-3710; (202) 777- APHA; TDD (202) 777-2500. APHA is a nongovernmental professional society founded in 1872, representing all disciplines and specialties in public health.

The *American Journal of Public Health*® (*AJPH*) (print ISSN: 0090-0036; electronic ISSN: 1541- 0048), first published in 1911, is the official journal of the American Public Health Association® (APHA). The oldest and largest organization of public health professionals in the world, APHA represents approximately 30 000 members from more than 50 occupations of public health.

Submissions: Visit www.editorialmanager.com/ajph or ajph.edmgr.com for online manuscript preparation and submission guidelines. Contributions of original unpublished research, social science analyses, scholarly essays, critical commentaries, departments, and letters to the editor are welcome. Questions? Write ajph.submissions@apha.org or call APHA at (202) 777-2469.

Print plus online subscriptions: Institutional price (print copy with online access for a single institution and all authorized users, regardless of geographic location) varies by size of organization and ranges from $993–$1445 for US organizations, and $1073–$1526 for international organizations (air delivery); multiple campuses not permitted without special arrangement. Details of the tiered pricing system at https://subscriptionoffice.com/pages/apha-landing-page. To order, write apha.subscriptions@apha.org.

Online-only subscriptions: Institutional price for one institution and its authorized users (regardless of geographic location) is $878–$1307. To order, write apha.subscriptions@apha.org. For academic consortia or multisite corporate subscriptions, contact apha.subscriptions@apha.org.

Print-only subscriptions: Institutional price is US $701, $782 international.

Back print issues: A limited number of print issues are for sale. Single copies are US $49, $55 international (air delivery). Shipping included; prepay only. To order, write apha.subscriptions@apha.org.

Reprints: For prices and ordering information on 50 or more reprints, check the Reprints section at www.ajph.org. To order smaller quantities of reprints (rush delivery), use the "Purchase Article" link on the article site itself.

Electronic access: Online articles more than 10 years old are available free for personal use at www.ajph.org. Recent articles are available through pay-per-view: single PDF article for $24, single issue access for 24 hours for $33, or entire site access for 24 hours for $38.

Postal information: Periodicals postage paid at Washington, DC, and additional mailing offices. Postmaster: Send address changes to American Journal of Public Health, 800 I St NW, Washington, DC 20001-3710.

Address changes: Send to AJPH, Membership Department (members) or AJPH Subscriptions (subscribers), APHA, 800 I St NW, Washington, DC 20001-3710. Or write to membership.mail@apha. org (members) or apha.subscriptions@apha.org (subscribers).

Advertising: For pricing and other information, see www.ajph.org. Please write to ashell.alston@apha.org or call (202) 777-2470 for other advertising opportunities. Ask about special exhibit packages and sponsorships. Acceptance of advertising by the *Journal* does not imply endorsement of products.

Indexes: Publications that index or abstract articles from AJPH include the following: Ageline, Assia (Applied Social Science Index and Abstracts), Biological Abstracts, Chemical Abstracts, CINAHL, Criminal Justice Abstracts, EMBASE, EMCare, Environmental Abstracts, e-psyche, ERIC, ETOH (Alcohol and Alcohol Problems Science Database), Excerpta Medica, Food Science and Technology, General Science Index, Grateful Med, Hospital Literature Index, Human Resources Abstracts, International Pharmaceutical Abstracts (IPA), Medline, Physical Education Index, Pollution Abstracts, Psychological Abstracts, PsychINFO, Safety Science Abstracts, Sage Family Studies Abstracts, Sage Human Resources Abstracts, Science Citation Index, SCOPUS, SIIC Data Bases, Social Work Research and Abstracts, and Statistical Reference Index (SRI)/LexisNexis.

AJPH

A PUBLICATION OF THE
AMERICAN PUBLIC HEALTH ASSOCIATION

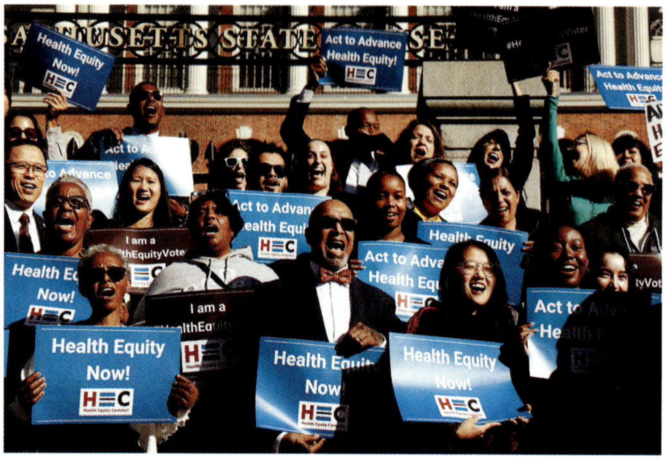

COVER: Craig Andrade, center, of the Boston University School of Public Health, joined in a chant during a rally organized by the Health Equity Compact, outside the Massachusetts State House. Following the rally the Joint Committee on Health Care Financing will hear testimonies from health system leaders and community members about the Health Equity Compact's bill, An Act to Advance Health Equity, a bill proposed to combat racial and ethnic health disparities in Massachusetts. The rally was organized by the Health Equity Compact, a group of more than 80 health leaders and experts.

Cover concept and selection by Aleisha Kropf. Photo by Craig F. Walker/ The Boston Globe via Getty Images. Printed with permission.

APHA
AMERICAN PUBLIC HEALTH ASSOCIATION
For science. For action. For health.

Promoting public health research, policy, practice, and education is the *AJPH* mission. As we widen our scope to embrace global issues, we also sharpen our focus to support the needs of public health practitioners. We invite contributions of original unpublished research, opinion and commentary, and letters to the editor.

The *Journal* is printed on acid-free recycled paper.

AJPH May 2024, Vol. 114, No. 5

OPEN ACCESS | ONLINE ONLY | PODCAST | DATA SUPPLEMENT AVAILABLE

EDITOR'S CHOICE

453 The *AJPH* Special Section on *The Future of Public Health*
P. C. Erwin

OPINIONS, IDEAS, & PRACTICE

EDITORIALS

455 Gender Identity and Ethnoracial Disparities in Conversion Effort Exposure
J. L. Turban, Chase T. M. Anderson, and J. Spetz

458 Is Law Enforcement Support the Missing Key to Thriving Syringe Service Programs in US Rural Areas?
S. M. Davis and A. L. Kristjansson

461 Our Public Health Workforce, Our Future: A Public Health of Consequence, May 2024
F. Kapadia

463 Looking Back: The Changing Landscape of Abortion Care in Louisiana
M. Pineda-Torres and Y. V. Rodgers

THE 1988 IOM REPORT

467 Celebrating 35 Years of Progress: The Past as Prologue to *The Future of Public Health*
H. H. Tilson

471 The 1988 IOM Report: A Philosophical Renaissance Short of Recommending a National Public Health System
C. W. Keck and R. Bialek

476 Our Catastrophe in Waiting: Climate Change
J. E. Fielding

479 Revisiting *The Future of Public Health*: The Good, the Bad, and the Ugly
R. C. Brownson and P. C. Erwin

486 Thirty-Six Years After the 1988 IOM *Future of Public Health*: Stop Ruminating and Start Taking Action
A. K. McGowan, S. Greeley, R. Griffis, and S. L. Polan

RESEARCH & ANALYSIS

THE 1988 IOM REPORT

489 The Influence of the 1988 and 2003 IOM *Future of Public Health* Reports on the CDC
E. L. Baker

495 Revisiting the IOM Reports and Envisioning a Promising Future for Public Health
A. B. Baciu and R. M. Martinez

CLIMATE CHANGE

501 Per- and Polyfluoroalkyl Substance Exposure Risks in US Carceral Facilities, 2022
L. Poirier, D. Salvatore, P. Brown, A. Cordner, K. Mok, and N. Shapiro

PERSPECTIVES FROM THE SOCIAL SCIENCES

511 Trajectories of Mental Distress Among US Women by Sexual Orientation and Racialized Group During the First Year of the COVID-19 Pandemic
A. L. Beccia, D. Zubizarreta, S. B. Austin, J. R. Raifman, J. E. Chavarro, and B. M. Charlton

SURVEILLANCE

523 Temporal Trends in Mental Health in the United States by Gender Identity, 2014–2021
D. Feir and S. Mann

OPEN-THEMED RESEARCH

527 State Medicaid Initiatives Targeting Substance Use Disorder in Criminal Legal Settings, 2021
C. D. Lewis, C. Andrews, A. J. Abraham, M. Westlake, F. S. Taxman, and C. M. Grogan

BACKMATTER

OTHER DEPARTMENTS

536 Subscription Form

The *AJPH* Special Section on *The Future of Public Health*

See also The 1988 IOM Report, pp. 461 and 467–500.

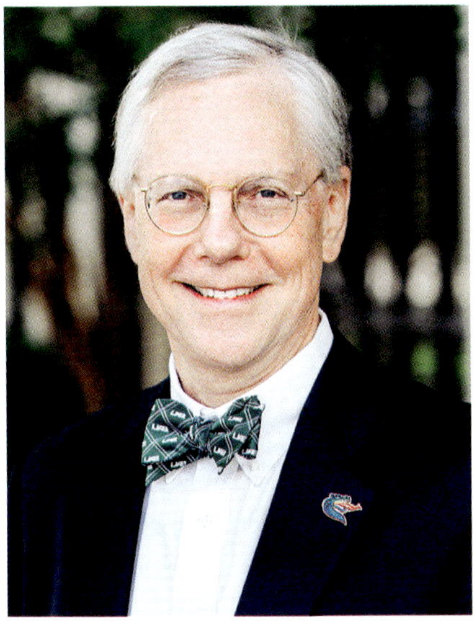

Paul C. Erwin, MD, DrPH
University of Alabama at Birmingham
AJPH Associate Editor

In 2023, *AJPH* issued a special call for articles on the impacts of the 1988 Institute of Medicine (now National Academy of Medicine) report *The Future of Public Health* (FOPH; https://bit.ly/3uX6l89) and the 2003 follow-up report *The Future of the Public's Health in the 21st Century* (FOPH21; https://bit.ly/3vdYent) on contemporary public health practice. We were interested in perspectives on the positive impacts of these reports, as well as the unintended consequences. Equally, we wanted to understand what system recommendations went unheeded and what recommendations were missing from these reports.

This special section begins with Tilson's editorial "Celebrating 35 Years of Progress: The Past as Prologue to *The Future of Public Health*" (p. 467), providing the history and context leading up to the 1988 FOPH report. As one of the very few surviving (and still very active!) original members of the Institute of Medicine Committee, Tilson's contribution is critical for future generations to understand why the FOPH work was needed, and thus why it produced the recommendations it did. Following this, Baker (p. 489) focuses on the many programs and activities that were either directly or indirectly a result of the FOPH and FOPH21 reports, with particular emphasis on the impact of the reports on the Centers for Disease Control and Prevention (CDC).

Shortcomings of the reports are pointed out by Fielding (p. 476), especially the inattention to the greatest public health threat we now face: climate change. Although the FOPH can hardly be faulted for that failure, as 1988 was the same year that NASA scientist James Hansen presented the first global warming models to Congress, FOPH21, published in 2003, completely missed this opportunity.

Brownson and I (p. 479) provide a report card on contemporary public health in light of the FOPH and FOPH21 reports and recommendations in describing the good (areas of significant progress), the bad (where progress is

Continued on page 454...

HISTORY CORNER

26 YEARS AGO

Creating the Future of Public Health

The future of public health is not in a crystal ball somewhere; it is not some pre-determined fate that we live out. Instead, as APHA Past President Dr Bill Foege often says, we create the future of public health together. We have the capabilities to create the future we want in our society-and, indeed, throughout the world. To accomplish this, we must engage the public in public health. . . . [A]s we move forward and create the future of public health together, let us remember the values that brought us into public health in the first place and not be afraid to articulate them, even in unfavorable political climates—to articulate them with passion, with courage, and with persistence.

From *AJPH*, February 1998, p. 189

32 YEARS AGO

The Future of Public Health

For all of the jubilant comparisons of health status today with morbidity and mortality trends in the early 1900s, most Americans now agree that serious impairments of the health services system persist. . . . These developments have injected such new urgency into the debate over the future of organized public health that the arguments for improving state and local public health services are no longer coming just from public health practitioners, health advocates, and the other usual proponents of community-oriented health and medical services. The business and industrial community-recognizing lagging), and the ugly (where there are strong warning signs and harms) in current public health practice. Calling for a shift in "our thinking about public health toward its value as a common good rather than a commodity," the editorial identifies several ideas for actions to address the "bad" and the "ugly."

McGowan et al. (p. 486), representing the American Public Health Association's recently established Alliance for Disease Prevention and Response, surmise that although the goals of the FOPH and FOPH21 reports were "laudable" and remain relevant and necessary, they are still largely aspirational. They report on the distillation of many recent reports and recommendations on improving the public health system—including The Bipartisan Policy Center's *Public Health Forward: Modernizing the US Public Health System* (https://bit.ly/43fOJAR), CDC Foundation's "Lights, Camera, Action" (https://bit.ly/4c7P7Fz), and The Commonwealth Fund Commission on a National Public Health System report, "Meeting America's Public Health Challenge" (https://bit.ly/43bWqYW)—and identify key lessons that will lead to action steps in the Alliance's Campaign for the Public's Health. Such lessons include the need to center communities in the work of public health, recognizing that the shift from health inequities to health equity will require a broader consideration of partnerships and an expansion of what we currently consider as the social determinants of health.

In Keck and Bialek (p. 471), current public health students can quickly see what they are learning across multiple courses: the 10 Essential Services, the Three Core Functions, the Academic Health Department, Public Health Performance Standards, and Public Health Accreditation, to name a few. Like Fielding and Baker, Keck and Bialek also identify shortcomings of the reports, including the failure to recommend a true national public health system.

Baciu and Martinez (p. 495) provide a current view on the two reports. (Note that both Baciu and Martinez served as Institute of Medicine staff on the FOPH21 Committee.) On the heels of the COVID-19 pandemic, their statement that public health is still in disarray because of insufficient and sporadic funding for public health functions and because of a lack of both public and policymaker awareness is particularly important given their organizational attachment. They highlight the numerous recent reports on the US public health infrastructure—similar to McGowan et al., as noted earlier—that not only underscore systems issues identified in FOPH and FOPH21 but reiterate the message that public health is more than the domain for governmental public health agencies. A call for a renewed focus on partnerships, including between public and private sectors and between public health practitioners and communities, suggests a path to better realizing the connections between democracy and health.

As one who began his public health career in 1988, in leading this special issue focus I am reminded of one of my favorite passages in "Little Gidding," the fourth of T. S. Eliot's *Four Quartets* (New York, NY: Houghton Mifflin Harcourt; 1943):

> We shall not cease from exploration
> And the end of all our exploring
> Will be to arrive where we started
> And know the place for the first
> time.

Yes, there is still much to celebrate in the FOPH and FOPH21 reports, and still work to be done for the next generations of public health academicians and practitioners. AJPH

DOI: https://doi.org/10.2105/AJPH.2024.307639

the value of comprehensive public health services to economic growth and development-calls for drastic improvements not just in schools and training programs but in water quality management, maternal and child health programs, and community nutrition services.

From *AJPH*, January 1992, pp. 21–22

34 YEARS AGO

Public Health's Promise for the Future

The public health enterprise has been greatly enhanced by the recent report of a comprehensive examination of its organization and practice. Considered a "landmark" study, the Institute of Medicine's (IOM's) report *The Future of Public Health* was completed and published in 1988. . . . The IOM report reinforces the importance of constituency building as a successful means of competing for resources and as a process for establishing policy priorities. Hence, fundamental to achieving the promise of public health is the establishment of reciprocal relationships with the public. This point was emphasized in a recent article on public hospitals. Using California as an example, the authors, Emmott and Wiebe, concluded that public hospitals as "safety nets" for the poor and uninsured are seriously threatened because they lack the resources to do the job. In their opinion, any short, intermediate or long-term reversal of resource allocations is dependent upon how successfully their urgency can be communicated to the public. . . . Public health advocacy in these matters and public health's ability to stimulate public support are important enhancement activities toward achieving its promise for the future.

From *AJPH*, August 1990, pp. 909–910

Gender Identity and Ethnoracial Disparities in Conversion Effort Exposure

Jack L. Turban, MD, MHS, Chase T. M. Anderson, MD, MS, and Joanne Spetz, PhD

ABOUT THE AUTHORS

Jack L. Turban is with the Division of Child and Adolescent Psychiatry, The Gender Psychiatry Program, and the Philip R. Lee Institute for Health Policy Studies at The University of California, San Francisco (UCSF). Chase T. M. Anderson is with the Division of Child and Adolescent Psychiatry, The MUSES Clinic, and The Gender Psychiatry Program at UCSF. Joanne Spetz is with the Philip R. Lee Institute for Health Policy Studies and the Department of Family and Community Medicine at UCSF.

Conversion efforts, sometimes referred to as "conversion therapies" or "reparative therapies," are attempts to force sexual and gender minority (SGM) people to be cisgender and heterosexual. They can be roughly delineated into sexual orientation conversion efforts (attempts to change a person's sexual orientation) and gender identity conversion efforts (attempts to change a person's gender identity); however, there is substantial overlap with these practices.[1]

Conversion efforts have been labeled dangerous and unethical by all major relevant professional organizations including the American Medical Association, American Psychiatric Association, American Academy of Pediatrics, American Psychological Association, and American Academy of Child and Adolescent Psychiatry.[2] They have been consistently linked to adverse mental health outcomes, including suicide attempts.[2–4] In addition to the mental health burden they create, they also have a substantial negative economic impact. A recent analysis estimated that, when associated harms such as substance use and suicide attempts were taken into account, conversion efforts had a total annual economic burden of $9.23 billion in the United States.[5] A recent independent expert report from the United Nations called for the practice to be banned worldwide.[4]

GENDER IDENTITY AND ETHNORACIAL DISPARITIES IN EXPOSURE

A new study by Tran et al.[6] adds yet another potential harrowing consequence of conversion efforts—exacerbation of ethnoracial and gender identity mental health disparities. The authors of this study used data, collected between 2019 and 2021, from more than 9000 participants from the Population Research in Identity and Disparities for Equality (PRIDE) study, a large nonprobability sample of SGM people in the United States. The survey included questions regarding lifetime exposure to conversion efforts, age of first exposure, and period of time between first and most recent exposure.

They found that 5.7% of participants overall were exposed to conversion efforts, and there were substantial disparities, with ethnoracially minoritized transgender and nonbinary (TNB) (prevalence ratio [PR] = 2.16; 95% confidence interval [CI] = 1.62, 2.86) and White TNB participants (PR = 1.57; 236; 95% CI = 1.30, 1.92) having greater prevalence of lifetime exposure when compared with White cisgender participants. Given the strong link between conversion effort exposure and adverse mental health outcomes, it is likely that these practices are contributing to the dramatic mental health disparities experienced by these populations. The results point to the need for continued research that will lead to targeted interventions to support each intersectional minoritized group.

THE US LEGAL AND POLICY LANDSCAPE FOR CONVERSION BANS

Despite the many deleterious consequences of conversion efforts, only about half of US states have banned the practice through legislation or executive order.[7] Increasingly, researchers are examining legal epidemiology (the study of how laws impact public health) and policy determinants of mental health among SGM people.[8] For instance, recent difference-in-differences causal inference analyses have linked state marriage equality laws to decreases in rates of suicidality among adolescents.[8] It has been hypothesized that the causal pathway of this relationship includes the implicit statement of social acceptance and support of SGM people, thus relieving stress that may be faced by SGM adolescents.[8] Conversely, laws permitting denial of services to SGM people have been found to cause an increase in adverse mental health outcomes.[8]

An implication of the study by Tran et al. is that conversion effort bans may mitigate the disparities in conversion effort exposure identified in their study. Other research has found benefits to conversion effort bans. For example, a recent difference-in-differences analysis linked conversion effort bans to decreases in rates of running away and suicidality among TNB individuals.[9] It is essential that clinicians and researchers continue to share relevant data with lawmakers and their constituents to promote evidence-based public policy, which has a dramatic potential to improve SGM mental health outcomes on a large scale. Public education campaigns with constituents may be particularly fruitful, as research has shown that state policymakers are less influenced by scientific data for health policy issues that have been similarly politicized (e.g., abortion policy and substance use during pregnancy policy).[10]

Another important finding from the study by Tran et al. is that the median age of first exposure to conversion efforts was 18.4 years. The high rates of exposure to conversion efforts during adulthood are made particularly clear by the study's Kaplan-Meier curve examining age of first exposure (Figure 1 in Tran et al.[6]). Unfortunately, most state bans on conversion efforts only cover minors, which may be insufficient to fully prevent the harms of this practice. Future public policies should consider banning this practice across the lifespan to protect public health.

Public health experts should also be aware of the evolving legal landscape regarding conversion effort bans. A recent decision from the US Court of Appeals for the Eleventh Circuit ruled that two conversion effort bans in Florida were unconstitutional because of their alleged infringement of free speech.[11] This perspective diverges from opinions from the US Courts of Appeals for the Third and Ninth Circuits, which upheld the constitutionality of similar bans, based on states' long history of regulating professional practice and states' interest in preventing dangerous practices by licensed professionals.[12] Given this circuit split, it is likely that the question may reach the US Supreme Court in the relatively near future.[12]

It will be helpful for researchers to examine some specific questions before the US Supreme Court takes on this question. When it comes to First Amendment analysis, it becomes important that laws be sufficiently "narrowly tailored" to achieve a state's interest (in this case, preventing the harms of conversion efforts). The decision from the Eleventh Circuit Court of Appeals raised concern that the Florida conversion effort bans were too broad, as they banned both aversive conversion efforts (e.g., shock therapies) and nonaversive conversion efforts (e.g., talk therapies).[11] The decision goes on to express concern that the negative impact of nonaversive conversion efforts specifically has not been adequately studied.[11] As with other past studies, this study by Tran et al. did not evaluate the modalities of conversion efforts to which people were exposed, an important area of focus for future research, so that this question can be answered for the courts. That being said, a strong argument could be made that the courts may concerningly ask for researchers to evaluate narrower and narrower subtypes of conversion efforts, which could create an impossible-to-reach scientific threshold.

CONCLUSION

As public health experts continue their work to identify the causes of and combat SGM mental health disparities, documenting the harms of conversion efforts and expanding the body of research related to their adverse impacts should continue to be prioritized. This new study by Tran et al. adds yet another reason that states have a compelling interest in banning conversion efforts—to combat gender and ethnoracial mental health disparities. As experts committed to improving public health, it is essential that we continue work to prevent these practices, given their dramatic adverse public mental health, economic, and health disparity impacts. AJPH

CORRESPONDENCE

Correspondence should be sent to Jack L. Turban, MD, MHS, Division of Child and Adolescent Psychiatry, University of California, San Francisco, 401 Parnassus Ave, San Francisco, CA 94143 (e-mail: jack.turban@ucsf.edu). Reprints can be ordered at https://ajph.org by clicking the "Reprints" link.

PUBLICATION INFORMATION

Full Citation: Turban JL, Anderson CTM, Spetz J. Gender identity and ethnoracial disparities in conversion effort exposure. *Am J Public Health*. 2024;114(5):455–457.

Acceptance Date: February 11, 2024.

DOI: https://doi.org/10.2105/AJPH.2024.307630

ORCID iD:

Jack L. Turban https://orcid.org/0000-0002-4877-254X

CONTRIBUTORS

All authors contributed to the conceptualization and outlining of this article. J. L. Turban wrote the initial draft, and all authors revised the article.

ACKNOWLEDGMENTS

This work was supported by R25 grant MH094612 from the National Institute of Mental Health (J. L. Turban), by The Sorensen Foundation (J. L. Turban), by the UCSF Population Health and Health Equity Scholars Program (J. L. Turban), and by The John A. Watson Scholarship from The UCSF School of Medicine Dean's Diversity Fund (C. T. M. Anderson).

CONFLICTS OF INTEREST

J. L. Turban reports receiving royalty payments from Springer Nature and Simon and Schuster and expert witness payments from the American Civil Liberties Union. He has previously received a Pilot Research Award for General Psychiatry Residents from the American Academy of Child and Adolescent Psychiatry, supported by industry donors (Arbor Pharmaceuticals and Pfizer).

REFERENCES

1. Ashley F. *Banning Transgender Conversion Practices: A Legal and Policy Analysis.* Vancouver, BC: UBC Press; 2022. https://doi.org/10.59962/9780774866941
2. Turban JL, Beckwith N, Reisner SL, Keuroghlian AS. Association between recalled exposure to gender identity conversion efforts and psychological distress and suicide attempts among transgender adults. *JAMA Psychiatry*. 2020;77(1):68–76. https://doi.org/10.1001/jamapsychiatry.2019.2285
3. Blosnich JR, Henderson ER, Coulter RW, Goldbach JT, Meyer IH. Sexual orientation change efforts, adverse childhood experiences, and suicide ideation and attempt among sexual minority adults, United States, 2016–2018. *Am J Public Health*. 2020;110(7):e1–e7. https://doi.org/10.2105/AJPH.2020.305637
4. Madrigal-Borloz V; United Nations Human Rights Council. Practices of so-called "conversion therapy": report of the Independent Expert on Protection Against Violence and Discrimination Based on Sexual Orientation and Gender Identity. 2020. Available at: https://digitallibrary.un.org/record/3870697?ln=en. Accessed January 29, 2024.
5. Forsythe A, Pick C, Tremblay G, Malaviya S, Green A, Sandman K. Humanistic and economic burden of conversion therapy among LGBTQ youths in the United States. *JAMA Pediatr*. 2022;176(5):493–501. https://doi.org/10.1001/jamapediatrics.2022.0042
6. Tran NK, Lett E, Flentje A, et al. Inequities in conversion practice exposure at the intersection of ethnoracial and gender identities. *Am J Public Health*. 2024;114(4):424–434. https://doi.org/10.2105/AJPH.2024.307580
7. Movement Advancement Project. Conversion "therapy" bans. 2024. Available at: https://www.lgbtmap.org/equality-maps/conversion_therapy. Accessed January 29, 2024.
8. Liu M, Turban JL, Mayer KH. The US Supreme Court and the future of sexual and gender minority health. *Am J Public Health*. 2021;111(7):1220–1222. https://doi.org/10.2105/AJPH.2021.306302
9. Campbell T, van der Meulen Rodgers Y. Conversion therapy, suicidality, and running away: an analysis of transgender youth in the US. *J Health Econ*. 2023;89:102750. https://doi.org/10.1016/j.jhealeco.2023.102750
10. Woodruff K, Roberts SC. "My good friends on the other side of the aisle aren't bothered by those facts": US state legislators' use of evidence in making policy on abortion. *Contraception*. 2020;101(4):249–255. https://doi.org/10.1016/j.contraception.2019.11.009
11. *Otto v City of Boca Raton*, 981 F3d 854 (11th Cir 2020).
12. The Associated Press. The Supreme Court rejects an appeal over bans on conversion therapy for LGBTQ+ children. 2023. Available at: https://apnews.com/article/supreme-court-lgbtq-conversion-therapy-ban-af3539f21f8618218b5029236182395d. Accessed January 29, 2024.

Is Law Enforcement Support the Missing Key to Thriving Syringe Service Programs in US Rural Areas?

Stephen M. Davis, PhD, and Alfgeir L. Kristjansson, PhD

ABOUT THE AUTHORS

Stephen M. Davis is with the Department of Health Policy, Management and Leadership, School of Public Health, West Virginia University, Morgantown. Alfgeir L. Kristjansson is with the West Virginia Prevention Research Center and Department of Social and Behavioral Sciences, School of Public Health, West Virginia University.

AJPH May 2024, Vol. 114, No. 5

A substantial body of evidence demonstrates the effectiveness of syringe service programs (SSPs) in preventing the transmission of infectious disease in people who inject drugs (PWID). The evidence is particularly strong with regard to HIV but is somewhat mixed for hepatitis C virus (HCV) unless an SSP is combined with opiate substitution therapy.[1] In a systematic review, Platt et al.[2] noted differences between Europe and the United States in the efficacy of SSPs for preventing HCV. In Europe, high SSP coverage was associated with a 76% reduction (risk ratio [RR] = 0.24; 95% confidence interval [CI] = 0.09, 0.62) in HCV incidence versus in North America, where no significant reduction was observed (RR = 1.25; 95% CI = 0.63, 2.46). Although selection bias and heterogeneity in the operationalization of intervention exposure may account for some of the observed continental difference, the authors point out the need to better understand variation in social, economic, and political factors on the two continents that may also affect SSP operations.

In the April 2024 issue of *AJPH*, Facente et al.[3] add to our understanding of the impact of SSP funding in the United States and the potential influence of social and political factors on funding levels. From their cross-sectional survey of SSPs operating in the United States between February and June 2022, the authors found that the median annual SSP budget of all programs was $100 000, which was more than $300 000 below the required estimated minimum costs of running a small (i.e., 250 clients) comprehensive SSP. Importantly, funding levels varied by urbanicity, with rural budgets meeting only 5% of the required operating costs compared with suburban and urban programs, which met 23% and 46% of the costs, respectively. Furthermore, Facente et al. found that SSPs operating in counties with a higher percentage of people voting Republican compared with other parties in the 2020 presidential election had significantly smaller operating budgets (adjusted mean difference = –$80 890). Although the authors acknowledge that further research is needed on the relationship between political orientation and SSP support, these observations are consistent with the experience in the majority Republican and rural state of West Virginia.

IMPORTANCE OF PUBLIC SUPPORT

The case of the Kanawha County Health Department SSP in Charleston, West Virginia, highlights how the role of public opinion can influence policy and, in this case, lead to the absence of available needs-based SSPs in a community. Briefly, in 2018, the Kanawha County SSP was shut down after its service to the community became a heated political issue, with some community leaders professing beliefs that the exchange promoted drug use, increased crime, and caused needle litter in public places.[4] After its closure, public health researchers noted increased risks of contracting HIV and HCV,[4] and HIV cases climbed over the next two years.[5]

The nearby city of Huntington in Cabell County, West Virginia, faced similar public backlash.[5] In an effort to keep its program open, a compromise was reached with local leaders[5] that involved a requirement for service users to show a form of identification and distribute syringes on a one-to-one basis, which is less effective than needs-based exchange.[4] Although the Centers for Disease Control and Prevention concluded that these restrictions contributed to an HIV outbreak,[6] many of these restrictions were adopted in a West Virginia law passed in April 2021.[4] This law included fines of up to $10 000 for programs violating any of the restrictions, thereby complicating already stretched SSP budgets.[7] Some existing syringe exchange programs in West Virginia closed after this law was enacted,[5,7] and at least one additional bill was introduced during the 2024 legislative session to make SSPs completely illegal in West Virginia.[8]

Public opinion reflected in the state legislature may, therefore, present an opportunity for health education on SSPs, with certain subgroups of the population likely to be more influential than others. One such group is law enforcement agents, who typically deal with PWID on a routine basis. Indeed, we have found that even if public policy permits SSPs with needs-based exchange, law enforcement support is a critical factor in maximizing SSP effectiveness.

KEY ROLE OF LAW ENFORCEMENT SUPPORT

Previously, we conducted a qualitative study with program directors, law enforcement agents, and PWID attending SSPs in West Virginia to determine the barriers and facilitators to using SSPs. A prominent theme in our findings was the legal conundrum created by paraphernalia laws that criminalize syringe possession and SSP provision of equipment to be used for illicit activities. This quandary contributed to confusion among many law enforcement agents and variable policing behaviors that resulted in some PWID being cited for possessing syringes, clean or used, that they had received from an SSP.[9] In a related quantitative study, we found that 72% of respondents cited fear of arrest as a key barrier to using a clean syringe during every injection.[10] Thus, the ability of SSPs to meet the public health goals of reducing infectious disease and overdoses likely is compromised in the absence of law enforcement support. However, the presence of law enforcement support transcends merely supporting the harm reduction goals of SSPs. Previous research has also shown that such support can facilitate the enactment of legislation authorizing syringe exchange in conservative areas.

In 2016, North Carolina became the first state with a Republican supermajority to pass legislation supporting SSPs.[11] Key to this legislation was the law enforcement community's appreciation of the harm reduction goals of SSP. Although somewhat contested, this appreciation was garnered through negotiating with and educating law enforcement personnel about the comprehensive services offered by SSPs and the fact that SSPs can minimize exposure to infectious diseases secondary to an accidental needlestick injury imposed on those in direct contact with PWID. The findings in North Carolina are consistent with our qualitative research in West Virginia[9] and with more recent work in rural areas of Kentucky.[12] However, law enforcement education alone may not be sufficient for legislative success. In the case of North Carolina, the SSP educational component helped secure the legislative support of a Republican sponsor who was a former chief of police.[11] Still, authorization for SSPs was negotiated and added only as an amendment to the main text of the bill, which restricted public disclosure of body camera footage.[13]

UNLOCKING SYRINGE SERVICE PROGRAM SUPPORT

Based on the experiences in Kentucky, North Carolina, and West Virginia, we suggest that future research focus on health education of law enforcement agents as a pathway to promoting the authorization and sufficient funding of SSPs in rural areas. However, research must also recognize the legislative and political trade-offs that may be required to secure SSP authorization. At a minimum this education should emphasize the shared goal of facilitating entry into treatment and the occupational health benefits of reducing exposure to bloodborne pathogens, both for PWID and law enforcement. Because law enforcement agents are important members of the public, especially in rural areas, they are in a prime position to influence opinions about SSPs among the general public, who may view syringe access as promoting illicit activity instead of keeping PWID safe with a goal of facilitating entry into treatment and reducing risks for those who serve them. Thus, garnering the support of law enforcement may be the key to unlocking higher SSP budgets, which Facente et al.[3] found to be associated with higher levels of syringe distribution and other harm reduction functions. AJPH

CORRESPONDENCE

Correspondence should be sent to Stephen M. Davis, PO Box 9190, WVU School of Public Health, 64 Medical Center Dr, HSC South, Room 3823, Morgantown, WV 26506-9190 (e-mail: smdavis@hsc.wvu.edu). Reprints can be ordered at http://www.ajph.org by clicking the "Reprints" link.

PUBLICATION INFORMATION

Full Citation: Davis SM, Kristjansson AL. Is law enforcement support the missing key to thriving syringe service programs in US rural areas? *Am J Public Health*. 2024;114(5):458–460.

Acceptance Date: February 27, 2024.

DOI: https://doi.org/10.2105/AJPH.2024.307647

CONTRIBUTORS

S. M. Davis drafted the editorial. A. L. Kristjansson provided important revisions to the editorial.

CONFLICTS OF INTEREST

The authors have no conflicts of interest to declare.

REFERENCES

1. Palmateer N, Hamill V, Bergenstrom A, et al. Interventions to prevent HIV and hepatitis C among people who inject drugs: latest evidence of effectiveness from a systematic review (2011 to 2020). *Int J Drug Policy.* 2022;109:103872. https://doi.org/10.21428/cb6ab371.e7a8b015
2. Platt L, Minozzi S, Reed J, et al. Needle and syringe programmes and opioid substitution therapy for preventing HCV transmission among people who inject drugs: findings from a Cochrane Review and meta-analysis. *Addiction.* 2018;113(3):545–563. https://doi.org/10.1111/add.14012
3. Facente SN, Humphrey JL, Akiba C, et al. Funding and delivery of syringe services programs in the United States, 2022. *Am J Public Health.* 2024; 114(4):435–443. https://doi.org/10.2105/AJPH.2024.307583
4. Hershow RB, Worthington N, Adams M, et al. A qualitative analysis of barriers to accessing HIV prevention services during an HIV outbreak among persons who inject drugs in West Virginia. *AIDS Behav.* 2024;28(2):669–681. https://doi.org/10.1007/s10461-023-04254-2
5. Kuehn BM. Restrictive policies threaten efforts to stop 2 West Virginia HIV outbreaks. *JAMA.* 2021;325(22):2238–2240. https://doi.org/10.1001/jama.2021.7404
6. Centers for Disease Control and Prevention. Notes From the Field: Outbreak of human immunodeficiency virus infection among persons who inject drugs—Cabell County, West Virginia, 2018–2019. *MMWR Morb Mortal Wkly Rep.* 2020;69(16):499–500. https://doi.org/10.15585/mmwr.mm6916a2
7. King Q. New W.Va. law forces another needle exchange closure. November 2, 2021. Available at: https://wvpublic.org/new-w-va-law-forces-another-needle-exchange-closure. Accessed March 6, 2024.
8. Weaver A. Some delegates want to prohibit needle exchange programs in West Virginia. January 17, 2024. Available at: https://www.wboy.com/news/west-virginia/west-virginia-politics/some-delegates-want-to-prohibit-needle-exchange-programs-in-west-virginia/#:~:text=(WBOY)%20%E2%80%94%20A%20bill%20introduced,saying%20syringe%20services%20are%20unlawful. Accessed March 6, 2024.
9. Davis SM, Davidov D, Kristjansson AL, Zullig K, Baus A, Fisher M. Qualitative case study of needle exchange programs in the central Appalachian region of the United States. *PLoS One.* 2018;13(10):e0205466. https://doi.org/10.1371/journal.pone.0205466
10. Davis SM, Kristjansson AL, Davidov D, Zullig K, Baus A, Fisher M. Barriers to using new needles encountered by rural Appalachian people who inject drugs: implications for needle exchange. *Harm Reduct J.* 2019;16(1):23. https://doi.org/10.1186/s12954-019-0295-5
11. Cloud DH, Castillo T, Brinkley-Rubinstein L, Dubey M, Childs R. Syringe decriminalization advocacy in red states: lessons from the North Carolina Harm Reduction Coalition. *Curr HIV/AIDS Rep.* 2018;15(3):276–282. https://doi.org/10.1007/s11904-018-0397-9
12. Allen ST, Danforth S, Grieb SM, et al. Law enforcement and syringe services program implementation in rural counties in Kentucky: a qualitative exploration. *Harm Reduct J.* 2022; 19(1):109. https://doi.org/10.1186/s12954-022-00684-8
13. Allen A. North Carolina legalizes needle exchange programs. July 12, 2016. Available at: https://mountainx.com/blogwire/north-carolina-legalizes-needle-exchange-programs. Accessed February 16, 2024.

Our Public Health Workforce, Our Future: A Public Health of Consequence, May 2024

Farzana Kapadia, PhD, MPH

ABOUT THE AUTHOR

Farzana Kapadia is AJPH *deputy editor, and professor of epidemiology, School of Global Public Health, New York University, New York.*

See also The 1988 IOM Report, pp. 453 and 467–500.

Every May, schools and programs of public health across the country hold commencement ceremonies that introduce a new cadre of public health professionals into the workforce. This is a time of both celebration of and reflection on the learning, both in the classroom and in practice-based settings (https://bit.ly/43rZIXS). These newly minted public health professionals will join or rejoin, as the case may be, the ranks of the public health workforce in academia; community-based settings; local-, state-, and tribal-level health departments; federal public health agencies; nonprofit and for-profit organizations; and private foundations. They will become public health practitioners and advocates, researchers, coordinators, nurses, doctors, social workers, and a whole host of other occupations that may not be readily evident as public health–related occupations.[1]

Against the backdrop of this achievement is the recognition that these graduates join the public health workforce during a crucial period. Understanding the current public health landscape that these graduates enter requires recognizing two types of force. First, since the 1988 release of the first IOM (Institute of Medicine; renamed National Academy of Medicine in 2015) report on the future of public health (https://bit.ly/3TcUpZ1), the public health workforce has been both a tool of and key to the evolution of public health infrastructure in the United States. Second, since the onset of the COVID-19 pandemic, those who graduate with a degree in public health are joining the workforce at a time when social, political, economic, technological, and environmental forces have coalesced to undermine trust in public health agencies and magnify failures while minimizing successes. Thus, the strides made in strengthening our public health workforce, the challenges that it faces moving forward, and efforts to overcome these challenges to secure our public health infrastructure merit reflection.

PUBLIC HEALTH WORKFORCE AS INFRASTRUCTURE

As summarized in several articles in this issue of *AJPH*, the 1988 and 2003 IOM reports marked dramatic evolutions in the conceptualization and strengthening of the public infrastructure across local-, state- and federal agencies. As noted by Baker (p. 489), the 1988 report laid the groundwork for reining in the "disarray" and "variability in the range of services provided by local health agencies across the nation" and moving toward a cohesive system of public health in the United States. By enumerating the three core functions and the 10 essential public health services, public health leaders were, in fact, documenting the range of services provided by public health workers—the bedrock of our entire public health system. Simultaneously, although they recognize public health workers as the foundation of all successful public health action, these early reports also identified the need for initiatives to enhance the technical as well as the leadership and management skills of the existing public health workforce. As noted by Gebbie during this time, the "current public health workers were originally hired for entry-level positions for which a specific skill was essential, and which did not require a general perspective."[2(p660)]

Since this time, several efforts at multiple levels have had varying effects on the professionalization of the public health workforce. For the earlier generation of public health employees, training and skills development coupled with leadership training were viewed as requisite for developing public health leaders. More recently, increases in undergraduate and graduate public health education have made inroads into strengthening the public health workforce.[3] However, these efforts alone will not ensure either our public health workforce or our public health enterprise. For graduates entering the public health workforce, sought after and desirable public health agencies will be those that offer competitive wages and benefits, productive working conditions (e.g., flexible work schedules), increased opportunities for career advancement and promotion, and greater employee empowerment.[4]

MODERN CHALLENGES FOR A MODERN WORKFORCE

Despite the progress and efforts in strengthening our public health workforce and agencies over these past 40 years, the events and movements of the past four years have clearly exacerbated gaps and inadequacies in our public health system. Public health graduates are emerging into a workforce that is being shaped, and hopefully reshaped, by the COVID-19 pandemic; the rise of the Black Lives Matter movement, which highlights the need to dismantle the deep-rooted structural racism that permeates our social systems; the climate change crisis; the opioid overdose epidemic; the gun violence epidemic; and the surge in mental health challenges facing adolescents. These issues call for public health workers to be able to take on bolder initiatives and collaborations to untangle the complex web of social determinants that influence health. Clearly, a public health workforce that is only able to promote a single program, intervention, or siloed effort to address a given health concern will not be able to achieve health equity and justice. Rather, bold thinking and bold solutions will be required to attain social justice and health equity.

OPPORTUNITIES AND SOLUTIONS

As summarized by Baciu and Martinez (p. 495), "Developments and innovations in cross-sector partnerships and the role of communities" show promise in moving the needle on achieving health equity. These are exactly the types of bold initiatives that have the potential to create synergies of positive impact across partner agencies and sectors to reduce barriers to accessing health care and related social services and drive structural change to promote health equity. To this end, and as described by Baciu and Martinez, our future public health workforce must have the understanding and skills, as well as be empowered to facilitate collaborations with private- and public-sector organizations and between partner agencies (e.g., housing, transportation), to enact the types of equitable solutions that can produce population-level benefits to health and well-being.

Baciu and Martinez also promote the integration of civic engagement in public health. Enabling community members to play an active role in using their resources to promote health equity and social justice will require active engagement in the political process. Whether via voting, volunteering, or grassroots community engagement, future public health professionals will need to be able to understand the political processes that shape public health policy. Moreover, they will need to be capable of capacity building in community organizations so that community members can become transformative agents in their own right.

Public health training has evolved to strengthen our public health institutions. Yet, what was previously done or is currently being done may not be what will work to secure our public health and well-being moving forward. Our public health workforce needs both training and power to develop and enact ideas—big and bold—to shape a public health system that works for all. AJPH

CORRESPONDENCE

Correspondence should be sent to Farzana Kapadia, PhD, MPH, New York University, School of Global Public Health, 708 Broadway, Room 729, New York, NY 10003 (e-mail: farzana.kapadia@nyu.edu). Reprints can be ordered at http://www.ajph.org by clicking the "Reprints" link.

PUBLICATION INFORMATION

Full Citation: Kapadia F. Our public health workforce, our future: a public health of consequence, May 2024. *Am J Public Health*. 2024;114(5):461–462.

Acceptance Date: February 22, 2024.

DOI: https://doi.org/10.2105/AJPH.2024.307644

CONFLICTS OF INTEREST

The author has no conflicts of interest to disclose.

REFERENCES

1. Krasna H, Venkataraman M, Robins M, Patino I, Leider JP. Standard occupational classification codes: gaps in federal data on the public health workforce. *Am J Public Health*. 2024;114(1):48–56. https://doi.org/10.2105/AJPH.2023.307463
2. Gebbie KM. The public health workforce: key to public health infrastructure. *Am J Public Health*. 1999;89(5):660–661. https://doi.org/10.2105/AJPH.89.5.660
3. Leider JP, Yeager VA, Kirkland C, et al. The state of the US public health workforce: ongoing challenges and future directions. *Annu Rev Public Health*. 2023;44:323–341. https://doi.org/10.1146/annurev-publhealth-071421-032830
4. Yeager VA, Wisniewski JM, Amos K, Bialek R. What matters in recruiting public health employees: considerations for filling workforce gaps. *Am J Public Health*. 2015;105(12):e33–e36. https://doi.org/10.2105/AJPH.2015.302805

Looking Back: The Changing Landscape of Abortion Care in Louisiana

Mayra Pineda-Torres, PhD, and Yana van der Meulen Rodgers, PhD

ABOUT THE AUTHORS

Mayra Pineda-Torres is with the School of Economics, Georgia Institute of Technology, Atlanta. Yana van der Meulen Rodgers is with the Labor Studies and Employment Relations Department, Rutgers University, New Brunswick, NJ.

Access to abortion, a health care service already long under siege from opponents, became even more tenuous as a result of widespread shutdowns and shelter-in-place orders during the COVID-19 pandemic. Service providers also experienced adverse effects, including shortages of personal protective equipment to ensure the safety of essential workers. COVID-19's introduction into an already restrictive landscape of abortion policies intensified the barriers that providers and communities faced, disproportionately impacting Black and Hispanic abortion seekers.[1]

In August 2021, Roberts et al. published a research article in *AJPH* showing that pandemic-related lockdowns and legal restrictions led to a 31% decline in the number of abortions per month in Louisiana but an increase in the likelihood of obtaining a second-trimester abortion.[2] In this editorial, we examine how COVID-19 and the *Dobbs* decision have impacted abortion services in Louisiana since the publication of this influential article. Concerns raised by Roberts et al. about the negative effects of clinic closures have only grown since their prescient study.

COVID-19–RELATED IMPACTS ON ABORTION SERVICES IN LOUISIANA

COVID-19 exacerbated the barriers people face in trying to access or practice abortion care. Across the country, social distancing requirements and the lack of childcare in the midst of school shutdowns placed limits on staffing capacity and the number of patients that clinics could schedule. Already experiencing a hostile legal environment before the pandemic, clinics in Louisiana faced additional threats as the state joined 12 others in designating abortion services as "nonessential" early in the pandemic.[3] Officials argued that restricting abortions would free up medical supplies and personnel by postponing elective procedures until the end of the crisis. The COVID-19 abortion bans were designed to reduce the number of abortions or force people out of state for abortion services, further adding to the monetary and time costs of obtaining an abortion.

Abortion is a time-sensitive service both in terms of health and in terms of legal restrictions. Forcing those who are pregnant to delay an abortion may endanger their physical health if the individual has a high-risk pregnancy or has complications from the procedure. Even though abortion is very safe, complications such as infection, hemorrhage, or uterine perforation are more common in second-trimester than first-trimester abortions.[4] Later or more complicated abortions are also more expensive and may entail more adverse mental health effects.[5] Delays could also extend the pregnancy to the point of fetal viability (designated as 20 weeks according to Louisiana law), after which most states prohibit abortions except to protect the life and health of the individual. The inclusion of abortion on the list of nonessential services was legally contested, with litigation in Louisiana and most other states resulting in abortion services remaining accessible.

Roberts et al. show that the monthly number of abortions requested by Louisiana residents in Louisiana clinics declined by 31% during the pandemic onset, with no evidence of an increase in out-of-state abortions that could compensate for this decline.[2] The timing of abortions also changed with the likelihood of a second-trimester abortion increasing. During the pandemic onset, Louisiana had only three open clinics, with only one or two of those having available appointments in any given month. This lack of service availability reflected a median wait time of more than two weeks, higher than in neighboring states. Louisiana also experienced a decrease in the proportion of abortions that were medication abortions (as opposed to aspiration abortion services), which the authors attribute to service availability in a facility that provided more aspiration than medication abortions. The relative decline may also be explained by the fact that Louisianans were forced to delay

AJPH May 2024, Vol. 114, No. 5

procedures (as demonstrated by the increase in second-trimester abortions), likely pushing them past the point at which medication abortion was an option.

Subsequent evidence in Berglas et al. indicates that Louisiana's decline in abortions, delay in abortion timing, and change in method were mainly concentrated among residents in areas where abortion care was disrupted.[6] Moreover, subsequent data released by the Guttmacher Institute indicate that the percentage of Louisiana residents obtaining abortions who traveled out of state increased from 13% in 2019 to 21% in 2020.[7] These studies show that Louisiana's pandemic abortion ban meaningfully disrupted people's ability to obtain abortions. As a result of the *Dobbs* decision, disruptions in abortion care have only worsened.

THE *DOBBS* DECISION AND REPERCUSSIONS FOR LOUISIANA

On June 24, 2022, the US Supreme Court overturned *Roe v Wade* and most aspects of *Planned Parenthood v Casey* in the case *Dobbs v Jackson Women's Health Organization*, which has left the legality of abortion up to the states. Before the *Dobbs* decision, most states had already implemented a series of state-level legal restrictions affecting both abortion seekers and providers, including parental consent for minors, targeted restrictions on abortion providers, mandatory pre-abortion counseling, pre-abortion waiting periods and testing requirements, physician-only laws, restrictions on medication abortion and telehealth, and insurance bans.

These restrictions resulted in clinic closures, fewer available appointments, and longer travel times and distances to obtain an abortion.[8–10] They also increased the monetary costs of abortion, which is already an expensive procedure and relatively difficult to finance for individuals with low incomes.[11] Federal and state restrictions on public funding for abortion costs, including the Hyde Amendment, further raised the out-of-pocket costs of abortions and increased the difficulty in accessing services for individuals with low incomes. Restrictions on private insurance plans that included abortion services had similar outcomes for abortion accessibility and costs. Abortion restrictions also adversely impacted child health, as shown in a comparison of individuals who received abortions with individuals who were denied abortions because of state regulations: people who were able to delay childbirth until they had greater economic and emotional security were able to raise their children in relatively better economic circumstances, with fewer indicators of delayed child development.[12]

The *Dobbs* decision allowed states not just to restrict abortion but also to ban abortion outright, even before viability. As of January 2024, abortion has been completely banned in 14 states, including Louisiana, and banned at an early gestational age in another two states. Note that several organizations have abortion law trackers, including the *New York Times*, Center for Reproductive Rights, Guttmacher Institute, and Kaiser Family Foundation. According to the Guttmacher Institute, Alabama, Arkansas, Idaho, Indiana, Kentucky, Louisiana, Mississippi, Missouri, North Dakota, Oklahoma, South Dakota, Tennessee, Texas, and West Virginia have all banned abortion, and Georgia and South Carolina have implemented six-week abortion bans.[13]

Many people must travel long distances to access abortion services. Nationally, the mean travel distance to access an abortion provider was 27.8 minutes before *Dobbs* and 100.4 minutes after *Dobbs*, with most of the additional time incurred by people living in and surrounded by ban states in the South and Midwest, especially Louisiana and Texas.[14] Before the *Dobbs* decision, 15% of reproductive-age women lived more than one hour away from an abortion provider; after *Dobbs*, that share rose to 33%.[14]

In Louisiana, the average distance to the nearest facility was 47 miles as of May 1, 2022.[15] However, a year later, in the wake of the *Dobbs* decision, the average distance for Louisiana residents increased to 456 miles—a 10-times increase in distance in one year (Figure 1). The state government further restricted access to abortion in June 2022 by making it a crime to receive mifepristone, the first of two drugs in a medication abortion, by mail, even though the US Food and Drug Administration had lifted restrictions on mailing mifepristone. As a result of the state's restrictive laws, Myers predicts a decrease in Louisiana's abortion rate of 29%[15] (unfortunately, data on post-*Dobbs* actual abortion rates for Louisiana are not available).

Louisiana residents have never experienced such a detrimental decline in access to abortion facilities as the one they are currently experiencing after *Dobbs*. Even during the COVID-19 pandemic, the average distance to the nearest abortion provider remained around 47 miles until the implementation of the state's abortion ban. In principle, people in Louisiana can obtain abortion services in other states. However, given the restrictive abortion landscape in neighboring states, distance

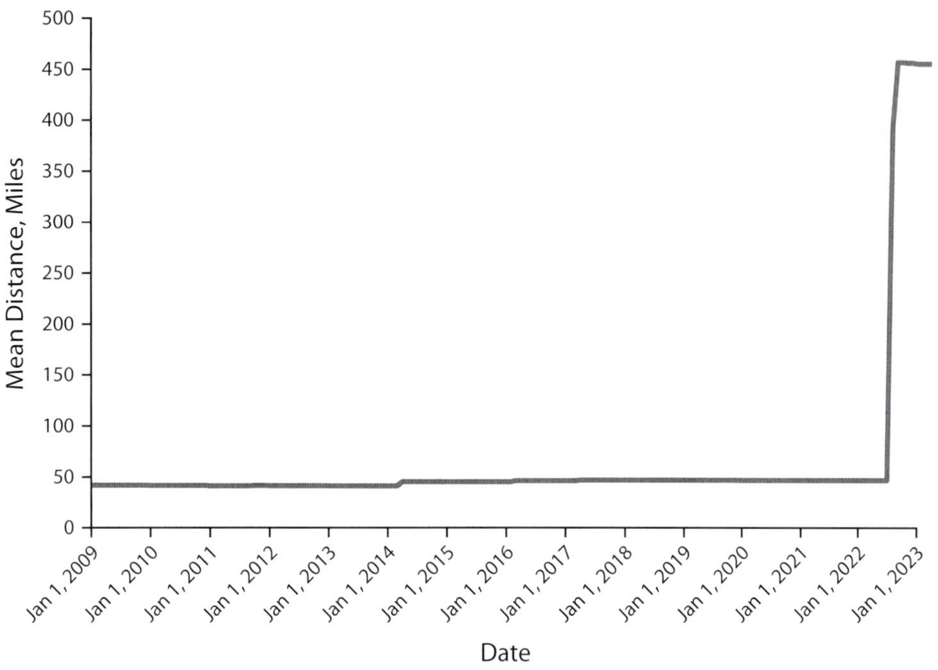

FIGURE 1— Average Distance From a County in Louisiana to the Nearest Abortion Facility: July 2021

Note. Our own elaboration using information on county-level distance to the nearest abortion facility from Myers.[16] The averages are weighted by the population of women aged 15 to 44 years in the origin county.

acts as a barrier to abortion, disproportionately affecting individuals with low incomes who lack the time and financial resources to travel out of state. This detrimental access to abortion is calculated to have "trapped" 23% of Louisianian abortion seekers and to have increased births by 3.2% in Louisiana during the first six months of 2023.[17]

MOVING FORWARD

Distance does not provide the complete picture of people's ability to obtain abortion services. After the *Dobbs* decision, every state showed a higher request rate of medication abortion from a telemedicine service involving a licensed provider, with the largest increase among abortion ban states.[18] Louisiana experienced the highest increase in weekly requests, from 5.6 per 100 000 female residents (in September 2021–May 2022) to 14.9 (in June–August 2022), even though Louisiana prohibits the use of telemedicine to provide medication abortions. Therefore, the inability to access abortion services has obliged abortion seekers to rely on self-managed abortion with pills obtained online outside of the formal health care system. Although self-managed abortion with pills can be medically safe and effective, it may not be an option for all Louisiana abortion seekers, given financial constraints and the legal risks of this alternative. Moreover, medication abortion, whether it be through a telemedicine provider or self-managed, is most effective early in pregnancy and may not be safe or effective for many later abortion-seekers.

A major political shift on abortion, at either the state or the federal level, is necessary but may take many years. In the meantime, relaxing existing restrictions on medication abortions and increasing advocacy efforts around eliminating legislative roadblocks to telemedicine delivery methods will go a long way to getting people the treatment they need. However, while expanding access to medication abortion is extremely important, some people will still require or prefer in-clinic care. The risk of avoiding a comprehensive shift in abortion law is a greater likelihood of individuals being unable to access facility-based care or to self-manage their abortions with pills; instead, they may use other methods that are ineffective and potentially unsafe.[19] Fewer restrictions on medication abortions will also support abortion providers doing this work by reducing the various risks they face, including exposure to the virus that causes COVID-19 and harassment at in-person clinics. Such measures have the potential to greatly reduce traditional racial, economic, and geographic barriers to abortion care. AJPH

CORRESPONDENCE

Correspondence should be sent to Yana Rodgers, 94 Rockafeller Road, Piscataway, NJ 08854 (e-mail: yana.rodgers@rutgers.edu). Reprints can be ordered at https://ajph.org by clicking the "Reprints" link.

PUBLICATION INFORMATION

Full Citation: Pineda-Torres M, Rodgers YV. Looking back: the changing landscape of abortion care in Louisiana. *Am J Public Health*. 2024;114(5): 463–466.

Acceptance Date: January 22, 2024.

DOI: https://doi.org/10.2105/AJPH.2024.307606

CONTRIBUTORS

The authors contributed equally to the conceptualization, writing, and editing of the article.

ACKNOWLEDGMENTS

The authors thank Mary Northridge, Alfredo Morabia, and Daniel Fox for the opportunity to contribute to *AJPH*'s Looking Back initiative, and they thank Elizabeth Sully, Jocelyn Finlay, and three anonymous reviewers for their helpful suggestions.

CONFLICTS OF INTEREST

The authors have no potential or actual conflicts of interest to declare.

REFERENCES

1. Wolfe T, Rodgers Y. Abortion during the COVID-19 pandemic: racial disparities and barriers to care in the USA. *Sex Res Social Policy*. 2022; 19(2):541–548. https://doi.org/10.1007/s13178-021-00569-8
2. Roberts SC, Berglas NF, Schroeder R, Lingwall M, Grossman D, White K. Disruptions to abortion care in Louisiana during early months of the COVID-19 pandemic. *Am J Public Health*. 2021;111(8):1504–1512. https://doi.org/10.2105/AJPH.2021.306284
3. Ruggiero S, Brandi K, Mark A, et al. Access to later abortion in the United States during COVID-19: challenges and recommendations from providers, advocates, and researchers. *Sex Reprod Health Matters*. 2020;28(1):1774185. https://doi.org/10.1080/26410397.2020.1774185
4. Grossman D, Blanchard K, Blumenthal P. Complications after second trimester surgical and medical abortion. *Reprod Health Matters*. 2008;16(suppl 31):173–182. https://doi.org/10.1016/S0968-8080(08)31379-2
5. Coast E, Lattof SR, Rodgers YV, Moore B, Poss C. The microeconomics of abortion: a scoping review and analysis of the economic consequences for abortion care-seekers. *PLoS One*. 2021;16(6):e0252005. https://doi.org/10.1371/journal.pone.0252005
6. Berglas NF, White K, Schroeder R, Roberts SC. Geographic disparities in disruptions to abortion care in Louisiana at the onset of the COVID-19 pandemic. *Contraception*. 2022;115:17–21. https://doi.org/10.1016/j.contraception.2022.07.012
7. Guttmacher Institute. Data Center. 2023. Available at: https://data.guttmacher.org/regions. Accessed October 10, 2023.
8. Fischer S, Royer H, White C. The impacts of reduced access to abortion and family planning services on abortions, births, and contraceptive purchases. *J Public Econ*. 2018;167:43–68. https://doi.org/10.1016/j.jpubeco.2018.08.009
9. Lindo JM, Myers CK, Schlosser A, Cunningham S. How far is too far? New evidence on abortion clinic closures, access, and abortions. *J Hum Resour*. 2020;55(4):1137–1160. https://doi.org/10.3368/jhr.55.4.1217-9254R3
10. Venator J, Fletcher J. Undue burden beyond Texas: an analysis of abortion clinic closures, births, and abortions in Wisconsin. *J Policy Anal Manage*. 2021;40(3):774–813. https://doi.org/10.1002/pam.22263
11. Lindo JM, Pineda-Torres M. New evidence on the effects of mandatory waiting periods for abortion. *J Health Econ*. 2021;80:102533. https://doi.org/10.1016/j.jhealeco.2021.102533
12. Foster DG, Biggs MA, Raifman S, Gipson J, Kimport K, Rocca CH. Comparison of health, development, maternal bonding, and poverty among children born after denial of abortion vs after pregnancies subsequent to an abortion. *JAMA Pediatr*. 2018;172(11):1053–1060. https://doi.org/10.1001/jamapediatrics.2018.1785
13. Guttmacher Institute. Interactive map: US abortion policies and access after Roe. Available at: https://states.guttmacher.org/policies. Accessed January 11, 2024.
14. Rader B, Upadhyay UD, Sehgal NKR, Reis BY, Brownstein JS, Hswen Y. Estimated travel time and spatial access to abortion facilities in the US before and after the Dobbs v Jackson women's health decision. *JAMA*. 2022;328(20):2041–2047. https://doi.org/10.1001/jama.2022.20424
15. Myers C. Forecasts for a post-Roe America: the effects of increased travel distance on abortions and births. *J Policy Anal Manage*. 2024;43(1):39–62. https://doi.org/10.1002/pam.22524
16. Myers CK. County-by-month distances to nearest abortion provider. Myers Abortion Facility Database. July 2021. https://doi.org/10.17605/OSF.IO/PFXQ3
17. Dench D, Pineda-Torres M, Myers CK. The effects of the Dobbs decision on fertility. IZA Discussion Paper No. 16608. November 15, 2023. SSRN 4634430. http://dx.doi.org/10.2139/ssrn.4636864
18. Aiken AR, Starling JE, Scott JG, Gomperts R. Requests for self-managed medication abortion provided using online telemedicine in 30 US states before and after the Dobbs v Jackson Women's Health Organization decision. *JAMA*. 2022;328(17):1768–1770. https://doi.org/10.1001/jama.2022.18865
19. Verma N, Grossman D. Self-managed abortion in the United States. *Curr Obstet Gynecol Rep*. 2023;12(2):70–75. https://doi.org/10.1007/s13669-023-00354-x

Celebrating 35 Years of Progress: The Past as Prologue to *The Future of Public Health*

Hugh H. Tilson, MD, DrPH

ABOUT THE AUTHOR

Hugh Tilson is with the University of North Carolina Gillings School of Global Public Health, Chapel Hill. He served on the panel that created the original Institute of Medicine report on the future of public health.

See also The 1988 IOM Report, pp. 453, 461, and 467–500.

The field of public health found much to celebrate when in June 2022 the Centers for Disease Control and Prevention (CDC) published the official request for applications for funding public health agencies and partners as part of implementation of the nation's American Rescue Plan Act of March 11, 2021 (Pub L No. 117-2). The CDC stated:

> COVID-19 has affected nearly every aspect of healthcare and public health, laying bare disparities and gaps in some conditions and worsening others. Public health agencies need the capacity to regain their footing in these areas and then accelerate their efforts.[1]

In the published announcement, the CDC further asserted:

> This funding is a first of its kind, noncategorical and cross-cutting [program] intended to help meet critical infrastructure and workforce needs in the short-term; and it should also make possible strategic investments that will have lasting effects on public health agencies across the United States. To that end, it will support strategically strengthening public health capacity and systems related to the workforce, foundational capabilities, data modernization, and support from national public health partners.[1]

To this member of the panel that produced the 1988 report of the Institute of Medicine (IOM) *The Future of Public Health*,[2] this legislation and its accompanying implementation also gave pause for reflection on how far we have come from the world of public health before 1988. The announcements represent the fulfillment of 35 years of work on the parts of thousands of colleagues (and friends) to implement the recommendations of that seminal 1988 report. Now we can take as givens what, in 1988, were only aspirations. It is now generally widely accepted that all communities must have the benefits of a local public health system, which is possible only if there is a local government component with essential services "which cannot be delegated"[2] (as urged in the 1988 report). It is axiomatic that these agents need to be trained and competent in the foundational capabilities of public health (then only being proposed in visionary descriptions of a model agency and aspirational suggestions for programs and services).

The current proposals clearly assume that all agree that proper surveillance and accountability require robust computer-based systems and trained statisticians and epidemiologists to work them, rather than trying to envision a world with better information collection and exchange (as described in the 1988 report). They describe roles and provide support for national public health partners, which were only strongly desired in 1988. And finally, of course, they offer noncategorical funding, recognized in 1988 as a critical and relatively absent tool for moving the public health effort forward.

PUBLIC HEALTH BEFORE 1988

To fully appreciate the enormity of this sea change since 1988, it might be helpful to review the state of public health that led up to the naming of the IOM committee. The runup to that landmark report was, curiously enough, also the result of inadequate pandemic preparedness, in that case, failures of our approach to the threatened epidemic of swine flu in 1976. Based on reports of a cluster of human-to-human transmission cases, the CDC activated the epidemic control plan and called for immediate and universal immunization of all US residents.

The public health community did what it could to respond, but it rapidly became apparent that the necessary systemic approach was not forthcoming. Some agencies (including the one for which I had responsibility at the time) were able to muster mass immunizations; far too many were not. Some were able to monitor and report; far too many were not. And when sporadic

AJPH May 2024, Vol. 114, No. 5

reports of Guillain-Barré syndrome emerged in association with the program, the nation's public health data systems were not robust enough to allow confirmation of whether the cases reflected excess prevalence (and hence a signal of a vaccine-related problem), leading to the inevitable fears and eventual abandonment of the national influenza vaccination effort. Mercifully, the anticipated pandemic did not materialize; sadly, that lucky turn resulted in adversarial posturing and accusations of crying wolf.[3]

MODEL STANDARDS AS A STEP FORWARD

Recognizing the clear evidence of the public health enterprise's inadequacy, in 1977, David Senser, then director of the CDC (who famously, or infamously, had injected then president Gerald Ford with swine flu vaccine on live TV), convened a panel of state and local public health practitioners and educators to propose a way forward to reframe the public health enterprise. To support the effort, a congressional mandate required us to develop model standards for community preventive health services. Over the intervening two years, the group labored long and hard to develop and publish a set of recommended metrics, which the CDC eventually published in 1978.[4] The model standards envisioned that every US community would have a public health presence that was able to assemble partners and agree on the state of health and health care in their community on an agreed-on set of benchmarks.

The process would entail an assessment of current shortfalls against desired expectations and result in an agreed-on set of plans and strategies for health improvement (essentially the precursor for what the public now takes as axiomatic: community health assessments and improvement plans). The model standards were a de facto workbook that included hundreds of proposed measures ("standards"), with a simple and consistent fill-in-the-blank format: "by 19xx, the rate of (condition yy) will not exceed (zz/1000)" or "by 19xx, the community will be served by a comprehensive system to address (condition yy)." In the absence of any precedent for what measures or efforts should be expected, standards were developed by nominal group process and chosen by leadership consensus.

LAUNCHING HEALTHY PEOPLE

In parallel, then surgeon general Julius Richmond, recognizing the urgent need for consensus on the goals and objectives that public health should be expected to address, issued a compelling surgeon general's report calling for agreement on the objectives to be expected from the nation's collective public health efforts.[5] Based on this report, the CDC launched the now decennial series of reports, the Healthy People program, with Healthy People 1990.[5] The first of the Healthy People reports, released in 1980, included 226 quantifiable objectives with proposals for targets to be achieved by 1990. The objectives were organized in the 15 priority areas identified in the 1979 surgeon general's report.

At the same time, the CDC supported a nationwide field test of the model standards, managed by the American Public Health Association (APHA; 1980–1982). After field testing for broader distribution, the APHA reconciled the model standards with the 1990 Healthy People objectives and republished them in 1985 as *Model Standards: A Guide for Community Preventive Health Services*, with the 1990 objectives as an appendix.[6]

The findings from this demonstration project were clear: in most settings where the application of the standards was attempted, the community found itself incapable of completing the process. Although the nation was moving toward consensus that public health should have specified and quantifiable objectives and agreed-on targets, these could not be readily translated into local action, where local infrastructure and data sets were insufficient. The nation did not have a public health delivery system capable of developing comprehensive strategies that align with the objectives even in the abstract, much less performing the services necessary for a coordinated community effort among system partners to achieve the proposed standards. Quite simply, the nation was incapable of mustering a concerted, aligned effort to ensure the urgently needed protections against major epidemics and other current and emerging public health challenges.

This failure should be seen in the context of many long-standing (but clearly insufficient) efforts to build an adequate public health enterprise. National advocates, notably the Association of State and Territorial Health Officials; the National Association of County Health Officials and its city counterpart, the US Conference of City Health Officers; and, of course, the APHA had robust campaigns to improve federal funding and organizational support for the state and local public health systems. Perhaps most notable were the successful efforts at the federal level for the creation of state and local comprehensive health planning agencies under the Comprehensive

AJPH May 2024, Vol. 114, No. 5

Health Planning and Public Health Services Amendments to the Public Health Service Act (Pub L No. 89–749; 1966) and its continuing amendments and improvements, particularly section 314(d), which permitted essentially no-strings funding of state and local public health agencies

> to enable the Surgeon General to make grants to state health or mental health authorities to assist the States in establishing and maintaining adequate public health services, including the training of personnel for State and local health work.[7]

Those witnessing the failures of the swine flu response and the subsequent efforts to build standards-based approaches to strengthen the public health enterprise were not surprised. However promising the preventive health services reform legislation, the appropriations were limited, their distribution was restricted, and many communities and essential services, much less public health infrastructure, were left unsupported.

ENGAGING THE IOM TO NAME THE "DISARRAY"

Armed with these dismaying findings, a small group from the public health leadership organizations involved in developing the model standards and Healthy People 1990 knew that it would take advocacy from the highest levels of national health policy to turn things around. They approached the National Academy of Sciences Institute of Medicine, the most prestigious among such national opinion leaders, and urged the development of a national level project at IOM to analyze the challenges and failures facing the nation's public health infrastructure. With organizational support and financing from the CDC, the Health Resources and Services Administration, and the Kellogg Foundation, IOM agreed and convened the blue-ribbon committee to study the future of public health.

With high-level, highly competent professional staffing led by IOM senior staffer Carl Yordy and a study panel led by distinguished dean of the University of Michigan School of Public Health, Richard Remington, that project, from 1986 to 1988, approached the public health enterprise with fresh eyes. They created an anthropological approach to analysis of the field, with site visits and public hearings to ask at state and local levels, "What is public health?" They invited participants to depict its scope and parameters, its strengths, limitations, and aspirations. In one most memorable site visit to a poor rural health department, when asked these questions by a site visit team, a county commissioner responded that public health in his community was "Whatever I say it is today." The watchword was "seen one health department, you've seen one health department." From the study, the inevitable conclusion was reached that the failures of the system that were all too visible after swine flu were widespread and profound. In short, the nation's public health enterprise was in disarray:

> This study was undertaken to address a growing perception among the Institute of Medicine membership and others concerned with the health of the public that this nation has lost sight of its public health goals and has allowed the system of public health activities to fall into disarray.[2]

Key among the findings was the realization that our nation lacked a universal agreement for the definition of the nature and scope of the field. Based on the work of the committee, the IOM recommended a new definition: that public health represents the collective efforts of society to fulfill "society's interest in assuring the conditions in which people can be healthy."[2]

The report then contrasted the current situation with this new aspirational definition:

> This report conveys an urgent message to the American people. Public health is a vital function that is in trouble. Immediate public concern and support are called for. . . . History teaches us that organized community effort to prevent disease and promote health is both valuable and effective. Yet public health in the United States has been taken for granted, many public health issues have become inappropriately politicized, and public health responsibilities have become so fragmented that deliberate action is often difficult if not impossible.[2]

Equally controversial were the findings that the educational institutions preparing the public health workforce had become "isolated from public health practice"[2] and that the vast majority of the public health workforce lacked, but needed, formal public health education. Finally, the report observed the vast gaps in distribution of services across the country and, most relevant to today's challenges, the urgent need to build and support a nationwide network of governmental public health agencies:

> Because of great diversity in size, powers, and capabilities of local governments, generalizations [about what a distributed official government public health infrastructure should look like] must be made with

> caution. Nevertheless, no citizen from any community, no matter how small or remote, should be without identifiable and realistic access to the benefits of public health protection, which is possible only through a local component of the public health delivery system.[2]

The report, in short, made the revolutionary call for a nationwide effort to provide the vision and mission of public health to deliver the system from disarray.[2]

The nation's leading medical opinion leader had spoken out. The long-standing struggle toward a rational distributed state and local public health infrastructure had been joined and the first steps on a vital new journey (now in its 35th year) taken. Tempting though it is to begin naming milestones along the march of 35 years to today's robust public health system—and tempting though it is to name some of the extraordinary, courageous, visionary leaders who have led or joined the march to bring about the embodiment of the vision of the 1988 report—let me leave those tasks to others.

The COVID-19 pandemic stretched all boundaries of preparedness and the public health infrastructure to unimaginable lengths. And yet we rose to and met the challenge, and we now have the obligation to take stock and move to the next level. As well documented in this issue of *AJPH*, although not in disarray, the system simply lacked adequate resources and systems to (fully) meet the challenges of the pandemic. The language of the request for application earlier referenced reflects this:

> The COVID-19 pandemic has emphasized the critical importance of a robust public health system. . . . Public health agencies need the capacity to regain their footing in these areas and then accelerate their efforts. This funding will . . . involve repositioning public health entities within the larger health and health care systems in which they operate. This will necessarily involve creating and strengthening partnerships at all levels. This program will also help to address the historic underinvestment in communities that are economically or socially marginalized, rural communities, and communities with people from racial and ethnic minority groups. This program also should support larger efforts to rebalance these investments and serve communities and populations that deserve more and better public health services.[1]

Thus, the words of the current CDC program announcement ring particularly true:

> Strengthen capacity and systems . . . build workforce . . . assure foundational capacities; . . . enhance data modernization . . . enlist national partners . . . advance health equity . . . support underserved communities.[1]

To those of us who were part of the landmark 1988 report, these words are music to the ears, every one of them an aspiration directly traceable to the recommendations of the 1988 report, then "visionary" but now "feasible" based on 35 years of progress. In short, *The Future of Public Health* is NOW! AJPH

CORRESPONDENCE

Correspondence should be sent to Hugh Tilson, University of North Carolina at Chapel Hill, Public Health Leadership, 525 Carolina Meadows Villa, Chapel Hill, NC 27517 (e-mail: Hugh_tilson@unc.edu). Reprints can be ordered at http://www.ajph.org by clicking the "Reprints" link.

PUBLICATION INFORMATION

Full Citation: Tilson HH. Celebrating 35 years of progress: the past as prologue to *The Future of Public Health*. *Am J Public Health*. 2024;114(5): 467–470.

Acceptance Date: October 23, 2023.

DOI: https://doi.org/10.2105/AJPH.2023.307520

CONFLICTS OF INTEREST

The author has no conflict of interests to report.

REFERENCES

1. Centers for Disease Control and Prevention. Strengthening US public health infrastructure, workforce, and data systems. June 2022. Available at: https://www.cdc.gov/workforce/resources/infrastructuregrant/pdfs/phi_grant_one_pager.pdf. Accessed February 27, 2024.
2. Institute of Medicine. *The Future of Public Health*. Washington, DC: National Academies Press; 1988.
3. Neustadt RE, Fineberg HV. *The Swine Flu Affair: Decision-Making on a Slippery Disease*. Washington, DC: National Academies Press; 1978.
4. US Conference of City Health Officers. *Model Standards for Community Preventive Health Services: A Report to the US Congress*. Washington, DC: Department of Health, Education, and Welfare; 1978.
5. *Healthy People: The Surgeon General's Report on Health Promotion and Disease Prevention*. Washington, DC: US Department of Health, Education, and Welfare; 1979.
6. American Public Health Association. *Model Standards: A Guide for Community Preventive Health Services*. Washington, DC; 1985.
7. Grants for Comprehensive Public Health Services, Pub L No. 89-749, Comprehensive Health Planning and Public Health Services Amendments, Section 314(d) (November 3, 1966).

The 1988 IOM Report: A Philosophical Renaissance Short of Recommending a National Public Health System

C. William Keck, MD, MPH, and Ron Bialek, MPP

ABOUT THE AUTHORS

C. William Keck is professor emeritus, Department of Family and Community Medicine, Northeast Ohio Medical University, Rootstown. Ron Bialek is president and CEO of the Public Health Foundation, Washington, DC.

See also The 1988 IOM Report, pp. 453, 461, and 467–500.

Over the past 35 years, the public health profession in the United States has undergone what has been characterized as a public health philosophical renaissance.[1] The primary progenitor of that renaissance was the seminal work by the Institute of Medicine (IOM) in its study of public health in the United States described in its 1988 report *The Future of Public Health*.[2] The famous conclusion in the report that governmental public health in the United States is a system in disarray was a call to action for the public health profession. The promise of comprehensive health reform made by President Clinton at the time of his election in 1992 provided additional stimulus for the public health community to respond enthusiastically to better define the role of public health, increase funding, and build public understanding of public health's contributions to health.

There ensued a period of unprecedented collaboration between agencies of the federal government; national public health professional organizations; state, tribal, local, and territorial health departments; and many individuals. This period was characterized by a strong sense of purpose and high productivity, resulting in such outcomes as a clear mission for public health, development of the 10 essential public health services, core competencies for public health professionals, national public health agency performance standards, clinical and community preventive services guidelines, a national public health research agenda, a public health code of ethics, and the development of public health leadership institutes.

We discuss some of the work done to strengthen academic–practice linkages since 1988 and describe how the absence of a financial and organizational renaissance to accompany its philosophical and workforce training gains continues to hamper the capacity of the public health profession. We also describe what is missing from the IOM reports, with further commentary on the work that remains unfinished.

THE PUBLIC HEALTH FACULTY–AGENCY FORUM

In response to the 1988 IOM report somewhat chastising schools of public health with its recommendation that "schools of public health should establish firm practice links with state and local health agencies,"[2(p157)] the Health Resources and Services Administration issued a request for proposals to establish a public health faculty–agency forum to explore ways that the practice and academic communities could work more closely together. The grant for establishing the forum was awarded in 1988 to the Johns Hopkins University School of Hygiene and Public Health[3] (the Centers for Disease Control and Prevention [CDC] provided additional funding later). Through the school's Health Program Alliance, one of the authors (R. B.) was the manager of this process, which brought an equal number of faculty and practitioners together to explore ways for the two communities to collaborate to advance the practice of public health.

Once the forum was convened, Bialek witnessed considerable animosity expressed between practitioners and faculty of schools of public health. One might speculate that a contributing factor to this animosity was the way the IOM reprimanded schools of public health. Much defensiveness was observed as practitioners reinforced the IOM's chastising remarks and faculty began discussing ways to increase the relevance to practice of public health education and research. In fact, one of the four forum workgroups considered not returning after the lunch break because the members of that group saw little, if any, opportunity to make progress on even recognizing each other's

AJPH May 2024, Vol. 114, No. 5

perspectives. Fortunately, this group did continue meeting and made progress on a key question: what do we want graduates of schools of public health to be skilled and competent in upon graduation?

When the forum completed its work a few years later, there was general agreement that there was a common set of skills and competencies that should apply to all public health professionals. This led to publishing the universal competencies for public health professionals in 1991.[3] The competencies have been regularly updated and were renamed the "core competencies for public health professionals."[4] They have been used as the foundation for discipline-specific competencies in many disciplines, including nursing, law, racial justice, and many public health specialties.[5] Once established, there was considerable discussion about how to implement these competencies and expand the role of schools of public health in initial education, continuing education, and research related to public health practice.

THE COUNCIL ON LINKAGES

Another important step for the forum was to develop recommendations and strategies that would lead to the use of the universal competencies and ways to better integrate the work of governmental public health agencies and schools of public health. Recommendations included linking academicians to practice by establishing required practicum experiences for master of public health students and fostering formal academic–practice partnerships. To implement these recommendations, the forum recommended the establishment of a "national steering committee on cooperation and collaboration" to promote and oversee implementation of the forum's recommendations.[3] The result was the creation of the Council on Linkages Between Academia and Public Health Practice (COL), with membership including the major governmental and public health professional organizations of the day (now totaling 24 members).[6]

As a convening and consensus-developing body, the COL members debated and developed different strategies for implementing the forum's recommendations. During its initial years, a strong consensus developed that it was desirable for all master of public health students to have a practicum experience to improve the practice relevance of public health curricula and tie educational institutions and tie practice agencies more closely together, an early recognition that the academic base for public health is much larger than just schools of public health. Discussions took place with the Council on Education for Public Health (CEPH), the accrediting body for schools and programs of public health, and ultimately CEPH adopted a practicum requirement. This requirement remains in place today and has resulted in all master of public health students of CEPH-accredited schools and programs receiving some practice experience before graduation.[7]

In 1984, following the example set by the 1974 Canadian Task Force on the Periodic Health Examination,[8] the US Public Health Service launched an effort to examine the effectiveness of clinical preventive services, resulting in the first of a number of subsequent publications titled *Guide to Clinical Preventive Services: An Assessment of the Effectiveness of 169 Interventions*.[9] In 1995, the COL thought a similar effort focused on community-based preventive services could strengthen the ties between academia and practice and help guide the practice of public health. This led to a W. K. Kellog Foundation grant for the COL to assess the desirability and feasibility of developing community preventive service guidelines and to test the methodology for evaluating scientific evidence for the effectiveness of community interventions. Practitioners and academicians collaborated to research potential practice guidelines, publishing one related to preventing the spread of tuberculosis through the use of directly observed therapy as an example of the kind of work that needed to be done.[10]

The results of this project were presented to the US Department of Health and Human Services assistant secretary for health and the director of the CDC. Agreeing that the COL had demonstrated both the desirability and the feasibility of developing evidence-based public health practice guidelines, the CDC created the Community Preventive Services Task Force to develop such guidelines.[11] This task force has been serving the public health community for more than two decades.

The COL also recognized the importance, for continuity's sake, of establishing more formal partnerships between individual practice and academic institutions. Often relationships across sectors are not formalized and depend more on personalities than any agreements being in place. This has led to the increasing desire of the COL, with encouragement from both practice and academia, to foster the development of mutually beneficial and formalized partnerships across the practice and academic sectors. The COL then created the Academic Health Department Learning Community in 2011.

Academic Health Department partnerships are defined as

> an arrangement between an academic institution and a governmental public health agency, which provides mutual benefits in teaching, research, and service, with academia informing the practice of public health, and the governmental public health agency informing the academic program.[12(p270)]

This learning community, staffed by the Public Health Foundation and now with approximately 1500 members, offers examples of Academic Health Department partnerships, two to four webinars per year addressing academic–practice partnership issues, sample partnership agreements, and other resources as well as exchanges of ideas and strategies through its listserv and at regional and national professional meetings.[13] This learning community continues to expand, with many successes of its members, including increasing capacity for providing public health services and assisting with accreditation efforts,[14] engaging in and translating research, applying for and receiving new funding, building skills and competence of students and faculty, placing students for internships and recruiting new staff,[15] and, most recently, responding to the COVID-19 pandemic (e.g., students engaging in contact tracing and faculty assisting with data analysis).[16]

THOUGHT AND ACTION EVOLUTION SINCE 1988

As understanding of the role of public health broadened at the end of the 20th century, it became increasingly clear that effectively addressing public health issues is an intersectoral responsibility. In 2003 the IOM issued the report *The Future of Public Health in the 21st Century*, which reviewed achievements and continuing vulnerabilities since its 1988 report.[17] In this report, it recognized the importance of providing student access to public health education in a broad range of disciplines now known to have a role in the maintenance and advancement of the public's health. It also called attention to the ongoing financial and infrastructure weaknesses in governmental public health and made recommendations for increased funding for infrastructure, legal reforms, and capacity building, among other things. It stopped short, however, of a recommendation to significantly reorganize governmental public health. The companion report, *Who Will Keep the Public Healthy?*, provided a framework and very specific recommendations for strengthening public health education, research, and practice.[18]

In the late 1990s, the Association of American Medical Colleges and the CDC established a cooperative agreement to strengthen collaborations between academic medicine and public health, recognizing that medical educators were struggling to integrate public health, population health, and prevention into medical curricula. A conference held in 2011 to share models and strategies that had been developed in this effort highlighted important progress made.[19] Despite some clear advances, in our opinion, this remains very much a work in progress today. As noted previously, public health competencies have been developed for a number of disciplines (e.g., nursing, law, racial justice), but little is known about their impact on curricula.

The 2013 decision by the Association of Schools of Public Health to open its membership to programs of public health and become the Association of Schools and Programs of Public Health increased the capacity of the organization to represent and advocate the needs of accredited public health education, service, and research. Programs that could afford the membership fee to join were brought into the mainstream and became more active participants in the evolution of public health training and its links to practice.

WHAT WAS MISSING FROM THE 1988 REPORT

Despite these clear successes, there were a few areas where the study committee's thinking was a bit narrower than it could have been. For example, the academic base for public health is much broader than the academic base for schools of public health. Graduate programs of public health also offer a variety of public health degrees, particularly the master of public health, and, as the IOM report noted, many other educational institution types (e.g., medicine, nursing, social work, health education, environmental health, mental health) produce graduates who end up working in governmental public health and community organizations. Improving the capacity of these institutions to prepare workers for public health practice is a valuable goal that goes beyond the capacity of just schools and programs of public health.

The 1988 IOM report also did not acknowledge that the way schools of public health are funded is not necessarily in line with promoting education and research for public health practice. However, the 2003 IOM report *Who Will Keep the Public Healthy?* addresses this issue, noting that public health education has been historically underfunded. Although the increase in National Institutes of

Health (NIH) funding for research strengthened quantitative disciplines, this further disadvantaged teaching and public health practice–oriented faculty.[18] The report further noted that despite some subsequent strengthening of ties between schools of public health and practice communities, an important remaining barrier is lack of funding and incentives for such activities. The incentive and reward structure for faculty tenure and promotion is weighted heavily toward research, with much less weight attached to teaching and practice activities.[18] On average, schools of public health derive approximately one quarter of their revenue from NIH funding.[20] Our continuing inability to come to grips with inadequate funding to prepare our public health workforce contributes to the professional "disarray" that remains today.

THE ELEPHANT IN THE ROOM

The 1988 IOM study committee did not include in its recommendations the development of a true national system of public health, or even suggest an agency or institution to fund and coordinate a nationwide response to their recommendations. The reality is that the public health profession in the United States is not organized into a system. For the most part, it consists of independent educational institutions and state, tribal, local, and territorial health departments tied together by a number of common goals and plagued by cyclical ebbs and flows of funding and unevenness in the distribution of resources. There is no national public health budget or administrative entity that can set universal goals and objectives for both education and practice, distribute resources as need dictates, or provide the necessary funding, planning, implementation, and evaluation processes.[21]

Despite the considerable progress that has been made to diminish disarray, the profession's inability to deal with the very politically fraught issue of developing a true national public health system leaves us with a ponderous mix of independent, large and small governmental public health agencies that vary widely in capacity and respond to no central authority[21] and workforce training that is inadequately supported.[17] The resultant independent governance and uneven distribution of talent and resources contribute to a continuing sense of disarray, especially when tested by a public health emergency, such as the recent COVID-19 pandemic.[22] Our unwillingness or inability to come to grips with this reality in both education and practice, with sporadic and inadequate funding often being a major contributing factor, significantly limits the likelihood that the ongoing identified weaknesses of governmental public health in this country will be well remedied.

CONCLUSIONS

The IOM's 1988 *The Future of Public Health* was a major contributor to understanding the issues beleaguering the public health profession 35 years ago and an important catalyst for the ensuing work that led to remarkable progress. In retrospect, we see that there are some issues that perhaps should have been addressed at that time, but many have been subsequently. In our view, however, despite progress made by efforts such as the public health faculty–agency forum and the COL, governmental public health agencies and workforce training institutions have insufficient capacity and coordination to respond to current and future population health needs with uniform excellence. To achieve this end, the profession's philosophical renaissance needs to be matched by a major funding and structural renaissance creating a true public health system. AJPH

CORRESPONDENCE

Correspondence should be sent to C. William Keck, MD, MPH, 3661 Bay Hill Dr, Fairlawn, OH 44333 (e-mail: keck@lek.net). Reprints can be ordered at http://www.ajph.org by clicking the "Reprints" link.

PUBLICATION INFORMATION

Full Citation: Keck CW, Bialek R. The 1988 IOM report: a philosophical renaissance short of recommending a national public health system. *Am J Public Health*. 2024;114(5):471–475.

Acceptance Date: February 8, 2024.

DOI: https://doi.org/10.2105/AJPH.2024.307624

CONTRIBUTORS

C. W. Keck combined the early drafts of the article and led the authors' responses to reviewer suggestions. R. Bialek made suggestions for changes and reviewed them before submission. Each author drafted a portion of the initial text, and both approve the final version to be published.

CONFLICTS OF INTEREST

The authors have no conflicts of interest to disclose.

REFERENCES

1. Scutchfield FD, Keck CW, eds. *Principles of Public Health Practice*, 3rd ed. Clifton Park, NY: Delmar, 2009.
2. Institute of Medicine, Committee for the Study of the Future of Public Health. *The Future of Public Health*. Washington, DC: National Academy Press; 1988.
3. Sorenson AA, Bialek RG. *The Public Health Faculty Agency Forum: Linking Graduate Education and Practice, Final Report*. Gainesville, FL: University Press of Florida; 1993.
4. Council on Linkages Between Academia and Public Health Practice. Core competencies for public health professionals. October 2021. Available at: https://www.phf.org/resourcestools/Documents/Core_Competencies_for_Public_Health_Professionals_2021October.pdf. Accessed February 27, 2024.
5. Centers for Disease Control and Prevention. Competencies for public health professionals. August 2023. Available at: https://www.cdc.gov/publichealthgateway/professional/competencies.html. Accessed February 27, 2024.
6. Public Health Foundation. Council on Linkages Between Academia and Public Health Practice. Available at: https://www.phf.org/programs/council. Accessed February 27, 2024.

7. Council on Education for Public Health. Accreditation criteria: schools and programs of public health. 2021. Available at: https://media.ceph.org/documents/2021.Criteria.pdf. Accessed February 27, 2024.
8. Canadian Task Force on the Periodic Health Examination. The periodic health examination. *Can Med Assoc J*. 1979;121(9):1193–1254. [Correction in: *Can Med Assoc J*. 1980;122(2):163].
9. US Preventive Services Task Force. *Guide to Clinical Preventive Services: An Assessment of the Effectiveness of 169 Interventions*. Baltimore, MD: Williams and Wilkins; 1989. https://doi.org/10.1016/S0025-6196(12)65716-4
10. Chaulk CP, Kazandjian VA. Directly observed therapy for treatment completion of pulmonary tuberculosis: consensus statement of the Public Health Tuberculosis Guidelines Panel. *JAMA*. 1998;279(12):943–948. https://doi.org/10.1001/jama.279.12.943
11. Truman BI, Smith-Akin CK, Hinman AR, et al. Developing the *Guide to Community Preventive Services*—overview and rationale. *Am J Prev Med*. 2000;18(1 suppl):18–26. https://doi.org/10.1016/S0749-3797(99)00124-5
12. Erwin PC, Keck CW. The Academic Health Department: the process of maturation. *J Public Health Manag Pract*. 2014;20(3):270–277. https://doi.org/10.1097/PHH.0000000000000016
13. Public Health Foundation. Academic Health Department Learning Community. Available at: https://www.phf.org/programs/AHDLC. Accessed February 27, 2024.
14. Public Health Foundation. Academic Health Department Learning Community meeting summary. December 8, 2011. Available at: https://www.phf.org/events/Pages/AHD_Learning_Community_Meeting_December_2011.aspx. Accessed February 27, 2024.
15. Public Health Foundation. Academic Health Department Learning Community meeting. January 16, 2016. Available at: http://www.phf.org/resourcestools/Documents/AHDLC_Jan2016_Meeting_Slides.pdf. Accessed February 27, 2024.
16. Pima County Health Department; University of Arizona. Academic Health Department webinar series: partners for public health. December 8, 2020. Available at: http://www.phf.org/events/Documents/AHD_Webinar_Slides_2020Dec.pdf. Accessed February 27, 2024.
17. Institute of Medicine. *Committee for the Future of the Public's Health in the 21st Century*. Washington, DC: National Academies Press; 2003.
18. Institute of Medicine. *Committee for Who Will Keep the Public Healthy?* Washington, DC: National Academies Press; 2003.
19. Maeshiro R, Koo D, Keck CW. Integration of public health into medical education: an introduction to the supplement. *Am J Prev Med*. 2011;41(4 suppl 3):S145–S148.
20. Freudenburg N, Klitzman S, Diamond C, El-Mohandes A. Keeping the "public" in schools of public health. *Am J Public Health*. 2015;105(suppl 1):S119–S124. https://doi.org/10.2105/AJPH.2014.302534
21. Wallace M, Sharfstein JM. The patchwork U.S. public health system. *N Engl J Med*. 2022;386(1):1–4. https://doi.org/10.1056/NEJM p2104881
22. Maani N, Galea S. COVID-19 and underinvestment in the public health infrastructure of the United States. *Milbank Q*. 2020;98(2):250–259. https://doi.org/10.1111/1468-0009.12463

Our Catastrophe in Waiting: Climate Change

Jonathan E. Fielding, MD, MPH, MBA

ABOUT THE AUTHOR

Jonathan E. Fielding is professor, Health Policy and Management, Fielding School of Public Health, and professor, Pediatrics, Geffen School of Medicine, University of California, Los Angeles.

See also The 1988 IOM Report, pp. 453, 461, and 467–500.

Two reports[1,2] of expert panels convened by the Institute of Medicine (IOM) to assess the state of public health were guided by the same mission statement: public health is what we can do as a society to assure the conditions in which people can be healthy. Going forward, what is our greatest opportunity to accomplish that mission and improve health at the population level?

THE FIRST REPORT

The first of these two reports,[1] released in 1988, was focused on the assessment of governmental public health agencies. It strongly suggested that insufficient investment in these agencies was largely responsible for inadequate progress in preventing and controlling diseases and injuries.

Widespread underfunding and fluctuating annual appropriations for state and local public health departments have contributed to variation in their capacity, effectiveness, and efficiency. But enhanced funding alone did not and will not eliminate major deficiencies in leadership, organizational structure, staffing, and experience.

We still live in a nation where the leading causes of mortality and disability are chronic diseases, such as cardiovascular disease, cancers, and mental health, and health-harming behaviors such as opioid use, smoking, unsafe driving, and deadly firearm injuries. Reducing these burdens requires close cooperation between many public agencies and private organizations. However, public health's traditional focus on disease and injury fails to address the serious underlying causes nor the major determinants of humankind's long-term well-being. Adding resources to governmental public health agencies to do more of the same, however necessary, is far from sufficient.

Thus, the charge to the 1988 report, *The Future of Public Health*,[1] left serious issues underaddressed. The report's title itself may have given readers the impression that our nation's efforts to improve health primarily work though state and local public health departments. The report did, however, recognize that public health's many collaborators, public and private, in health care, mental health, and, importantly, in other sectors, needed to address our collective health were identified. Unfortunately, the resources required for public health to do so were not forthcoming. Moreover, since it was US-focused, there was no discussion of what we could learn from public health agencies in other high-income nations with better health outcomes.

THE SECOND REPORT AND *HEALTHY PEOPLE*

The second IOM report, entitled *The Future of the Public's Health in the 21st Century*,[2] was published in 2002, almost 15 years after the first. At first glance, it appeared to maintain the definition of public health in the 1988 report. However, closer examination revealed a strategically placed apostrophe S modifying "Public" in the title. That small orthographic change emphasized a broader scope, encompassing all public and private organizations whose actions affect health at the population level. The second report was strongly influenced by *Healthy People 2010*,[3] released in 2000 by the US Department of Health and Human Services, which filled in some detail suggested by the 1988 report. It proposed a comprehensive national agenda with 467 objectives to increase years of healthy life and to eliminate health disparities. It outlined a systems approach to assuring the nation's health in practice, research, and policy. That document further emphasized the critical role of nongovernmental entities in all sectors via strategic partnerships.

Multiple broad determinants of our collective health and ill health—social, economic, and political environments—were a central theme of *Healthy People 2010*[3] and the second IOM[2] report. Critical emphasis was accorded variations in health status, termed "disparities," on the path to more accurately brand them as "inequities." The rapidly increasing disconnect between health care cost expenditures and population health was also highlighted.

Some noteworthy improvements in the public's health have occurred since the IOM reports; however, there are also many lessons from our collective failures to ameliorate some burdens of ill health. After years of progress in extending lifespan, from 1977 to 2019, our rank in longevity dropped from 14th to 46th among 236 other countries.[4] But worse, much worse, is yet to come no matter what actions we take now. We know that because the inciting conditions are already baked into our environment.

A MAJOR GAP

While the 1988 report was written as critical information was just emerging, the subsequent IOM report, several iterations of *Healthy People* and many public health leaders have in common that we were missing in action for too long in identifying the most important issue we will ever confront and for which our inaction will be called out as, at best, ignorant, and, more properly, tragic, threatening our entire civilization—climate change.

How could public health ignore this singular existential threat to *Homo sapiens* as a species for multiple decades? Despite the period between 1940 and 1970 when global temperatures declined slightly because of a higher release of sunlight deflecting aerosols, virtually all the experts in atmospheric chemistry and related disciplines have found a clearcut causal relationship between rising atmospheric carbon and global warming, beginning with the start of the Industrial Revolution. Indeed, 2023 was the hottest year on record. Ironically, many experts consider 1988, the year of the first IOM report, as a turning point. That summer was the hottest on record and was accompanied in the United States by extensive wildfires and drought. That same year, NASA scientist James Hansen[5] presented models to Congress relating that he was 99% sure that we were suffering from global warming.

Implications of the expert models of increasing global warming were many: exceptional heat, intensive storms, extended droughts, increasing wildfires, accelerated melting of glaciers with sea level rise of between 11 and 38 inches by 2100,[5] and increased communicable diseases. All the experts, except a few supported by fossil fuel producers, agreed that greenhouse gases from burning fossil fuel were the cause of climate change and the singular existential threat to a habitable planet. Efforts to reduce the global release of greenhouse gases to limit global warming to at least 1.5 degrees Centigrade (2.7 degrees Fahrenheit) ensued internationally, starting with the 1997 adoption of the Kyoto Protocol,[6] and subsequent international treaties setting goals for nations to limit greenhouse gases. Yet many signatory nations are falling below their promised reduction targets under the current Paris Accord.[7]

Where was our public health enterprise in this history? Did we sound the alarm that climate change is the greatest threat to our collective health? Did we reprioritize our work accordingly? Did we brief the elected officials on what we and our sister organizations could do in support of a smaller carbon footprint? Did we expose the disinformation of the fossil fuel companies, who were using the tobacco company playbook to instill doubt that climate change was real and that disastrous consequences were already baked into the current greenhouse gas concentration?

Like many city, county, and state leaders, I was late to the fray. I only started to talk about the effects of climate change already in evidence in about 1995 and only become a committed climate change fighter after reading about the scientific consensus and the dire predictions. As Los Angeles County public health officer and department head, I resolved to build the capacity to sound the alarm broadly and develop departmental expertise in how best to adapt to worsening heat-related health and environmental problems and support efforts to mitigate the concentration of carbon dioxide (CO_2) and other greenhouse gases.

But I had to fight with the county bureaucrats who did not see the need or value in hiring an expert in climate change. Fortunately, our environmental health chief and our science officer were forward-thinking leaders with high credibility. Together we prevailed and in 2010 formed a climate change unit headed by a PhD in environmental health. That unit has become the coordinating resource for all departments in developing policies and programs for Los Angeles County, the most populous county in the United States.

The two IOM reports also failed to mention, much less emphasize, population growth as a major contributor to climate change. From 1800 to present, world population increased from an estimated 1 billion to about 8 billion, with reasonable projections of an additional 2 billion over the next 30 years. The maximum carrying capacity of the planet is unknown, but if we have not already exceeded it, we are currently at high risk because of inadequate food supply, dwindling water reserves, and environmental degradation.

One obvious reason for a slow public heath response was the disinformation campaign funded by the fossil fuel industry, which succeeded in getting many politicians, including two American presidents, to deny the science-supported link between increased atmospheric CO_2 and global warming.

Why, then, was this overriding issue still not given prominence in the second IOM report? In many states and locales, environmental issues are the purview of a separate department and, often, public health agencies are cautioned to "stay in their own lane." And most state and local health departments lack expertise in climatology and environmental epidemiology. That must be rectified.

As public health has embraced the broader concepts of population health, it is imperative that public health leaders develop the expertise and vision to place climate change at the top of our action agenda. The public is beginning to see the concrete impacts of climate change on their lives with wildfires, hurricanes, drought, floods, and heat domes. As the health effects become more salient, public health must give voice to the human toll and promote near- and long-term solutions. We owe it to future generations to leave them a habitable planet. AJPH

CORRESPONDENCE

Correspondence should be sent to Jonathan E. Fielding, MD, MPH, MBA, UCLA Pub Hlth-Hlth Policy & Mgmt, BOX 951772, 61-253 CHS, Los Angeles, CA 90095-1772 (e-mail: jfieldin@ucla.edu). Reprints can be ordered at https://ajph.org by clicking the "Reprints" link.

PUBLICATION INFORMATION

Full Citation: Fielding JE. Our catastrophe in waiting: climate change. *Am J Public Health*. 2024; 114(5):476–478.

Acceptance Date: December 21, 2023.

https://doi.org/10.2105/AJPH.2024.307575

ACKNOWLEDGMENTS

Thank you to Steven Teutsch for assistance in preparation of this article.

CONFLICTS OF INTEREST

The author has no conflicts of interest to disclose.

REFERENCES

1. Institute of Medicine Committee for the Study of the Future of Public Health. *The Future of Public Health*. Washington, DC: National Academies Press; 1988.
2. Institute of Medicine Committee on Assuring the Health of the Public in the 21st Century. *The Future of the Public's Health in the 21st Century*. Washington, DC: National Academies Press; 2002.
3. US Department of Health and Human Services. *Healthy People 2010*. Available at: https://www.cdc.gov/nchs/healthy_people/hp2010.htm. Accessed January 17, 2024.
4. Woolf SH. Falling behind: the growing gap in life expectancy between the United States and other countries, 1933–2021. *Am J Public Health*. 2023; 113(9):970–980. https://doi.org/10.2105/AJPH.2023.307310
5. Intergovernmental Panel on Climate Change. Special Report on the Ocean and Cryosphere in a Changing Climate. Summary for Policymakers. 2019. Available at: https://www.ipcc.ch/srocc/chapter/summary-for-policymakers. Accessed January 17, 2024.
6. United Nations Climate Change. Kyoto Protocol - Targets for the first commitment period. Available at: https://unfccc.int/process-and-meetings/the-kyoto-protocol/what-is-the-kyoto-protocol/kyoto-protocol-targets-for-the-first-commitment-period. Accessed January 17, 2024.
7. United Nations Climate Change. The Paris Agreement. What is the Paris Agreement? Available at: https://unfccc.int/process-and-meetings/the-paris-agreement. Accessed January 17, 2024.

Revisiting *The Future of Public Health*: The Good, the Bad, and the Ugly

Ross C. Brownson, PhD, and Paul C. Erwin, MD, DrPH

ABOUT THE AUTHORS

Ross C. Brownson is with the Prevention Research Center at the Brown School and the Division of Public Health Sciences and Alvin J. Siteman Cancer Center, School of Medicine, Washington University in St Louis, MO. Paul C. Erwin is an AJPH associate editor and is with the School of Public Health, University of Alabama at Birmingham.

See also The 1988 IOM Report, pp. 453, 461, and 467–500.

We began our careers in public health practice around the time of the release of the landmark 1988 report, *The Future of Public Health* (FOPH).[1] Perhaps the most widely publicized quote in the report was "this nation has lost sight of its public health goals and has allowed the system of public health to fall into disarray."[1(p1)] The FOPH highlighted the fragmented and non-interconnected public health system, along with public complacency. While the theme of disarray was the attention getter, many other topics have resonated in the intervening 35 years, showing the prescience of the FOPH, including the introduction of core functions of public health, the central role of science, and ongoing gaps in workforce development.

Many others have expanded upon and critiqued the FOPH report. Critiques included a lack of a national vision and too much emphasis on site visits to six states.[2] Largely missing was a central focus on health equity, particularly a focus on historical structural drivers of inequities.

Multiple other reports from the Institute of Medicine covered related themes, including a 2003 report that focused on a policy approach to population health, the need to emphasize broader determinants of health, the power of partnerships, and the need for systems to address accountability and communication.[3] Three related committees reviewed population health strategies, metrics, and interventions[4]; how statutes and regulations can optimize health outcomes[5]; and recommendations for funding state and local health systems.[6]

We provide our current snapshot of public health in light of the 1988 FOPH report and those that followed—we assess where we are making significant progress ("the good"), where progress is lagging ("the bad"), and where there are strong warning signs and harms ("the ugly"). Because we allocate more space to what needs more attention, our inclusion of "the good" will be brief.

THE LEDGER ON PROGRESS

Against the backdrop of macro trends affecting public health (e.g., big data, shifting demographics, climate change)[7,8] and the "fault lines" (e.g., inadequate surveillance, lack of investment in public health, lack of public trust) revealed by COVID-19,[9,10] we offer a report card on multiple issues being faced by public health. Some of these were directly addressed in the FOPH report, whereas others were alluded to or only indirectly discussed, and still others were not even imagined in 1988 (e.g., workplace violence against public health employees).

The Good

Investment in the public health workforce. At the time of the d schools of public health and eight accredited programs of public health in the United States; as of July 31, 2023, there were 64 accredited schools, 149 accredited programs, and 27 accredited standalone baccalaureate programs in the United States.[11] Although this phenomenal growth in academic programs could be seen as an expanded pipeline for public health practice workforce development, this is not fully apparent in national databases such as the Public Health Workforce Interests and Needs Surveys (PH WINS).[12] In 2021, PH WINS showed that only 14% of state and local governmental public health employees had a public health degree.

Accreditation of public health agencies. The 1988 FOPH report recommended standards, minimum services, and methods of financing for local public health functions.[1] This report and the work of multiple other groups led to the establishment of a national voluntary program for public health agency accreditation through the Public Health Accreditation Board (PHAB) in 2007. As of July 31, 2023, PHAB had accredited 41 state, 321 local, and six tribal public health agencies.[13] There is growing evidence of the impact and value of accreditation,[14] including an association

AJPH May 2024, Vol. 114, No. 5

between PHAB accreditation and evidence-based decision-making.[15]

Emphasis on the linkages between public health practice and academia. A significant aspect of the "disarray" of public health in the FOPH report was the disconnect between governmental public health agencies and academic institutions, particularly schools of public health.[1] One of the first important responses to this academic–practice disconnect was the establishment of the Public Health Faculty/Agency Forum as a means for translating the Institute of Medicine's recommendations on the engagement between academia and public health practice.[16] This work eventually led to the development of the "academic health department" concept, first described by Keck,[17] with subsequent significant expansion of engagement between practitioners at both the state and local level and academicians as described by the Academic Health Department Learning Community.

Rise of implementation research. The importance of implementation research was mentioned multiple times in the FOPH, mainly because it provides a set of research methods to bridge academia and public health practice. Implementation research seeks to understand the processes and factors that are associated with successful integration of evidence-based interventions (EBIs) within a particular setting (e.g., a worksite or school).[18] A broader interpretation of implementation research also includes the study of discontinuation of interventions and practices that do not work or uptake of underutilized EBIs (de-implementation[19] and mis-implementation[20]). These concepts are especially important for making the best use of limited resources in public health, resulting in more efficient policy choices. Over the past several years, implementation research has placed a stronger focus on health equity, with an urgency to improve the speed and reach of EBIs to marginalized communities.[21–23]

Growth of evidence-based public health. While the FOPH report did not explicitly describe the term "evidence-based public health" (EBPH), it highlighted in multiple places the science underlying public health and many important tools for following an evidence-based process. Following landmark publications on evidence-based medicine in the early 1990s,[24] the movement to establish the tenets of EBPH took hold in the late 1990s.[25–27] The core principles of EBPH include making decisions based on the best available scientific evidence, using data and information systems systematically, applying program planning frameworks, engaging the community in decision-making, conducting sound evaluation, and disseminating what is learned.[28] The EBPH movement has benefitted greatly by the increased availability of a broad menu of EBIs.[29–31]

Focus on equity and social risks. Finally, one area that the FOPH report did not focus on, but for which there has been something "good" subsequent to the report, is health equity. Over the 35 years since the report, there has been an increasing emphasis and urgency to address health equity, driven by several factors including increases in income inequality[32] and the visibility and impacts of historic structural racism.[33] Viewing public health practice with a health equity lens moves away from a deficit mindset of what society is doing poorly (disparities) to one that is positive about what society can achieve (equity).[34] Public health agencies are taking stronger roles in addressing health equity in multiple ways, including making health equity a core value of the agency, building skills among staff members, and developing systems to track health equity progress.

The Bad

Retention and salaries among practitioners. The FOPH report noted that the average tenure of a state health officer was two years, while the median salary of the "principal state health official" (in 1987) was approximately $55 000 ($134 000 in today's dollars). The authors went on to note that not only did low pay make it difficult to recruit and retain leaders, but inadequate salaries also fed into the negative image of public health practice.

In the 2014 PH WINS, nearly one in five state health department employees indicated they were planning to leave their job within one year,[35] and 40% of survey respondents reported being somewhat or very dissatisfied with their pay. By the 2021 PH WINS, conditions had worsened: nearly one third of state and local public health employees (32%) said they were considering leaving their organization in the next year,[36] and almost half of those planning to leave gave low pay as the leading reason.

Role of policy-based evidence. The focus on policy development was clearly evident in the FOPH report; however, the report had much less to say about evidence-based policy. For a wide range of public health interventions, the return on investment is large and is often highest for policy approaches.[37] Evidence-based policy decisions are grounded in, or influenced by, rigorous objective evidence. Kingdon notes very distinct "streams" that, when co-occurring, increase the odds of a policy being adopted.[38] The first of these is the evidence of the problem. The second is the development of potential policies to solve that problem. Finally, there is the role of politics, factors both inside and outside of government that influence policymaking. Policy change occurs when a "window of opportunity" opens and policy actors align the three streams to push through evidence-based policy change.

Policy-based "evidence" is the reverse process—instances in which a policymaker has already decided what they want to do and then searches for evidence to support their position,[39] often for ideological and political purposes. This has become particularly problematic during the COVID-19 pandemic. In studies of US local elected officials, policymakers who were ideologically predisposed against a policy were relatively unwilling to learn from others, but such ideological biases can be overcome with framing of the policy's success or adoption of the policy by copartisans in other communities.[40]

Rising inequities. Despite a growing focus on health equity—part of the "good" in public health practice[34]—more urgency, greater political will, and new approaches are needed. In recent data tracking of progress toward achieving *Healthy People 2020* objectives, inequities by race and ethnicity were reduced in only 20 of the 505 (4%) health objectives since its launch in 2010.[41] The necessity to address equity is also illustrated by declining US life expectancy among subgroups. For example, among the American Indian/Alaska Native population, life expectancy was 65.2 years in 2021, a decrease of 6.6 years since 2019 and the same life expectancy as the total US population in 1944.[42] In mapping life expectancies in several cities across the United States, there are differences as large as 20 years in neighborhoods just a few miles apart.[43] The United States has the highest geographic health disparities among 11 high-income countries.[44]

The Ugly

Politicization and polarization in public health. Public health has always been political.[45] The FOPH report discussed the dynamics of US politics and how these forces can make progress in public health difficult. On the heels of COVID-19, public health is perhaps more politicized than ever before, and this increasing politicization is part of the larger forces that are impacting trust in government. The politicization of public health is closely connected to the polarization of the electorate. Polarization occurs when population subsets take on dissimilar attitudes toward political parties and party members (affective polarization) as well as ideologies and policies (ideological polarization).[46] Polarization and politicization also both contribute to, and are influenced by, the epidemic of misinformation that has been experienced throughout the pandemic.

Progress in public health requires policies supporting health—reaching policy consensus is more difficult in a politicized and polarized society. In a study of US residents, Fraser et al. found consistent patterns that individuals who feel more politically different from the average voter in their state reported more days of poor health outcomes.[47] The long-term challenge for public health officials is convincing political leaders to view their efforts as a health practice, not as something always viewed through a political lens.[48] This may be easier at the local level, where trust in local government may facilitate effective communication with elected officials and residents.

Harassment of public health workers. The 1988 FOPH did not imagine outright workplace violence affecting governmental public health employees. A strong influence on public health employees' decisions to leave governmental public health agencies has been the direct negative effects of COVID-19 on the workforce. In a media content analysis and a national survey of US local health departments, there were nearly 1500 individual instances of workplace violence against public health officials between March 2020 and January 2021.[49] Partly as a result of these experiences, 10% of state and local health departments experienced a loss or departure of leadership, with a third directly attributable to harassment. The share of US adults who believed that harassing or threatening public health officials because of business closures was justified rose from 20% to 25% and 15% to 21%, respectively, from November 2020 to July and August 2021.[50]

From the 2021 PH WINS of local health department employees, there are high levels of stress and burnout among the public health workforce. More than half of all public health employees reported one or more symptoms of posttraumatic stress disorder, and 25% reported three or more symptoms, equating to probable posttraumatic stress disorder. Forty percent of public health workers, especially leaders, reported bullying, threats, and harassment.

Assault on human rights. Human rights is a necessary condition for advancing social justice and a central foundation for public health policies and programs.[51] The focus on human rights as international law began with the Universal Declaration of Human Rights in 1948.[52] The declaration established that everyone has a right to an adequate living standard for the health and well-being of the individual and family. In the United States, civil rights laws have been essential in extending protections and privileges to multiple groups, including individuals from racial and ethnic minority groups, women, people with disabilities, and lesbian, gay, bisexual, transgender, and queer (LGBTQ) individuals.[53] Public health should address rights related to equity, nondiscrimination, and participation of marginalized groups.[54]

Despite advances, human rights face unprecedented threats in the United States, largely because of the emergence of the populist radical right.[51] For example, voting is the centerpiece of democracy—it shapes the public health landscape in multiple ways. Voting is consistently associated with health—individuals with poorer health outcomes are less likely to engage in voting—and gaps in voting may be associated with electoral outcomes.[55] Yet, voting rights are under challenge in the United States because of policy actions to restrict access to voting.[56] Second, a record number of anti-LGBTQ bills have been introduced over the past few years in state legislatures.[57] These bills will cause harm to LGBTQ people in civil rights, health, education, and public accommodation.

SUMMARY AND A WAY FORWARD

Society at large and policymakers can become complacent about public health—taking it for granted when it is working at its best (the invisibility of prevention) and criticizing public health during a crisis. We need to shift our thinking about public health toward its value as a common good rather than a commodity.[58] For each of the "bad" and "ugly" issues noted, we provide a brief summary, ideas for actions, and selected resources (Box 1).

BOX 1— Ways of Addressing Core Public Health Challenges (the "Bad" and the "Ugly")

Challenge	Core Issues	Actions to Address	Selected Data Sources and Resources
Retention and salaries among practitioners	• Low salaries among governmental public health professionals are a challenge for recruitment and retention. • More than one third of state health department employees plan to leave within five years.	• Show the real-world impacts of the work of (nonelected) public health practitioners. • Identify creative ways of increasing the salary structure for practitioners. • Develop agency-specific plans for retention and replacement of workers who retire or move to a different job. • Review human resource practices in governmental public health agencies. • Adjust public health curricula to prepare and inspire students for governmental public health.	PH WINS https://debeaumont.org/phwins/what-is-phwins Partnership for Public Service https://ourpublicservice.org
Policy-based evidence	• Policymaker seeks out evidence to support a position already determined.	• Three "streams" are important (problem, policy, politics). • Policy change happens when a window aligns with the three streams. • Fund and implement systematic tracking of policies (i.e., policy surveillance). • Translate empirical evidence into easily understood stories. • Align evidence, if available, with priorities of the policymaker. • Engage with copartisans in other communities (nongovernmental organizations, private sector).	Center for Evidence-based Policy https://centerforevidencebasedpolicy.org National Conference of State Legislatures https://www.ncsl.org Center for Public Health Law Research https://phlr.org Evidence-Based Policymaking Resource Center https://www.pewtrusts.org/en/research-and-analysis/articles/2018/12/18/evidence-based-policymaking-resource-center

Continued

BOX 1— Continued

Challenge	Core Issues	Actions to Address	Selected Data Sources and Resources
Rising inequities	• Life expectancy is declining in some racial/ethnic subgroups. • The United States has the highest geographic health disparities among high-income countries. • Inequities are highly influenced by structural drivers (racism, unequal access to housing and education).	• Show the value and impact of EBIs that address health equity and social determinants. • Better balance health needs and social needs in marginalized populations. • Conduct more disease- and risk factor–agnostic interventions. • Enhance skills in working across sectors and agencies outside of health. • Provide structural interventions in collaboration with other sectors (housing, education) to address drivers.	Building a Movement, Transforming Institutions: A Guide for Public Health Professionals https://www.policylink.org/our-work/community/health-equity/institutionalizing-health-equity Pathways to Population Health Equity https://www.publichealthequity.org
Politicization and polarization in public health	• Public health may be more politicized than ever. • Politicization is closely connected with polarization of the electorate. • Trust in governmental public health agencies has declined. • Trust is higher at local and state levels than at the national level. • Misinformation is a significant challenge for public health.	• Educate elected leaders to view public health as a practice, not a political activity. • Reach the electorate on public health issues via a variety of channels (social media, local meetings, mass media). • Disseminate information via nonpartisan experts and coalitions. • Identify "super-spreaders" of misinformation. • Enlist trusted community members to address public health issues where misinformation is common. • Provide as much transparency as possible in governmental actions. • Recommit governmental public health agencies to solving big problems. • Empower citizen voice in governmental decision-making. • Rebuild trust in science-based public health through clear messaging.	National Conference of State Legislatures https://www.ncsl.org National Governors Association https://www.nga.org Partnership for Public Service https://ourpublicservice.org Open Government Partnership https://www.opengovpartnership.org Confronting Health Misinformation https://www.hhs.gov/sites/default/files/surgeon-general-misinformation-advisory.pdf Community Toolkit for Addressing Health Misinformation https://oes.gsa.gov/collaborations/misinformation-toolkit
Harassment of public health workers	• Harassment of public health workers is common. • One quarter of public health workers report three or more symptoms of posttraumatic stress disorder.	• Establish a reporting system for incidents of violence against public health workers. • Provide legal protections for public health workers. • Work with coalitions and elected officials to protect the statutory authority of public health.	Stop Harassment and Violence https://standwithpublichealth.jhsph.edu/stop-harassment-against-workforce The Network for Public Health Law https://www.networkforphl.org
Assault on human rights	• Human rights is a central pillar for public health. • Human rights face unprecedented threats. • Many topics and groups are at risk (e.g., voting rights, reproductive rights, LGBTQ populations).	• Establish human rights as a core function of public health. • Join forces between public health practitioners and advocates to address human rights.	World Health Organization: Human Rights https://www.who.int/news-room/fact-sheets/detail/human-rights-and-health Human Rights Watch https://www.hrw.org/topic/health The Carter Center https://www.cartercenter.org

Note. EBI = evidence-based intervention; LGBTQ = lesbian, gay, bisexual, transgender, and queer; PH WINS = Public Health Workforce Interests and Needs Survey.

Our job as public health professionals is to identify, advocate, implement, and evaluate practices and policies that will improve health. Progress begins with adequate investment—we vastly underinvest in public health, and public health funding from all sources (governmental, private) has declined over the past several decades.[59] We also need to train practitioners with the skill sets to prepare them for future challenges, not for the issues and technologies of the past.[7,60]

The science underlying public health (e.g., a suite of EBIs) has grown exponentially since the publication of the landmark FOPH report—yet we have not fully harvested these advances and marshalled the political will to advance equity and population health. AJPH

CORRESPONDENCE

Correspondence should be sent to Ross C. Brownson, Washington University in St Louis, One Brookings Dr, Campus Box 1196, St Louis, MO 63130 (e-mail: rbrownson@wustl.edu). Reprints can be ordered at https://ajph.org by clicking the "Reprints" link.

PUBLICATION INFORMATION

Full Citation: Brownson RC, Erwin PC. Revisiting *The Future of Public Health*: the good, the bad, and the ugly. *Am J Public Health*. 2024;114(5):479–485.

Acceptance Date: December 4, 2023.

DOI: https://doi.org/10.2105/AJPH.2023.307558

CONTRIBUTORS

R. C. Brownson conceptualized the original essay and wrote the draft of the article. P. C. Erwin provided input on the original outline, contributed text to the draft article, and provided critical intellectual content to the article. Both authors approved the final version.

ACKNOWLEDGMENTS

This work was supported in part by the National Cancer Institute (P50CA244431), the National Institute of Diabetes and Digestive and Kidney Diseases (P30DK092950), the Centers for Disease Control and Prevention (U48DP006395), and the Foundation for Barnes-Jewish Hospital.

Note. The findings and conclusions in this article are those of the authors and do not necessarily represent the official positions of the National Institutes of Health or the Centers for Disease Control and Prevention.

CONFLICTS OF INTEREST

The authors have no conflicts of interest to disclose.

REFERENCES

1. Institute of Medicine. *Committee for the Study of the Future of Public Health. The Future of Public Health.* Washington, DC: National Academy Press; 1988.
2. Annas GJ, Glantz LH, Scotch NA. Back to the future: the IOM report reconsidered. *Am J Public Health.* 1991;81(7):835–837. https://doi.org/10.2105/AJPH.81.7.835
3. Institute of Medicine. *The Future of the Public's Health in the 21st Century.* Washington, DC: National Academies Press; 2003.
4. Institute of Medicine; Committee on Public Health Strategies to Improve Health. *For the Public's Health: The Role of Measurement in Action and Accountability.* Washington, DC: Institute of Medicine of The National Academies; 2010.
5. Institute of Medicine; Committee on Public Health Strategies to Improve Health. *For the Public's Health: Revitalizing Law and Public Policy to Meet New Challenges.* Washington, DC: Institute of Medicine of The National Academies; 2011.
6. Institute of Medicine; Committee on Public Health Strategies to Improve Health. *For the Public's Health: Investing in a Healthier Future.* Washington, DC: Institute of Medicine of The National Academies; 2012.
7. Brownson RC, Samet JM, Chavez GF, et al. Charting a future for epidemiologic training. *Ann Epidemiol.* 2015;25(6):458–465. https://doi.org/10.1016/j.annepidem.2015.03.002
8. Erwin PC, Brownson RC. Macro trends and the future of public health practice. *Annu Rev Public Health.* 2017;38(1):393–412. https://doi.org/10.1146/annurev-publhealth-031816-044224
9. Brownson RC, Burke TA, Colditz GA, Samet JM. Reimagining public health in the aftermath of a pandemic. *Am J Public Health.* 2020;110(11):1605–1610. https://doi.org/10.2105/AJPH.2020.305861
10. Narayan KMV, Curran JW, Foege WH. The COVID-19 pandemic as an opportunity to ensure a more successful future for science and public health. *JAMA.* 2021;325(6):525–526. https://doi.org/10.1001/jama.2020.23479
11. Council on Education for Public Health. Accredited schools and programs. Available at: https://ceph.org/about/org-info/who-we-accredit/accredited. Accessed July 31, 2023.
12. de Beaumont Foundation. What is PH WINS? Available at: https://debeaumont.org/phwins/2021-findings/#phwins-resources. Accessed July 31, 2023.
13. Public Health Accreditation Board. The National Voluntary Accreditation Program. Available at: http://www.phaboard.org. Accessed August 2, 2023.
14. Public Health Accreditation Board. *The Value and Impact of Public Health Department Accreditation.* 2023. Available at: https://phaboard.org/wp-content/uploads/PHAB-Value-and-Impact.pdf. Accessed February 29, 2024.
15. Erwin PC, Padek MM, Allen P, Smith R, Brownson RC. The association between evidence-based decision making and accreditation of state health departments. *J Public Health Manag Pract.* 2020;26(5):419–427. https://doi.org/10.1097/PHH.0000000000001162
16. Erwin PC, Grubaugh JH, Mazzucca-Ragan S, Brownson RC. The value and impacts of academic public health departments. *Annu Rev Public Health.* 2023;44(1):343–362. https://doi.org/10.1146/annurev-publhealth-071421-031614
17. Keck CW. Lessons learned from an academic health department. *J Public Health Manag Pract.* 2000;6(1):47–52. https://doi.org/10.1097/00124784-200006010-00008
18. Rabin B, Viglione C, Brownson R. Terminology for dissemination and implementation research. In: Brownson R, Colditz G, Proctor E, eds. *Dissemination and Implementation Research in Health: Translating Science to Practice.* 2nd ed. New York, NY: Oxford University Press; 2023:27–68.
19. McKay VR, Morshed AB, Brownson RC, Proctor EK, Prusaczyk B. Letting go: conceptualizing intervention de-implementation in public health and social service settings. *Am J Community Psychol.* 2018;62(1-2):189–202. https://doi.org/10.1002/ajcp.12258
20. Brownson RC, Allen P, Jacob RR, et al. Understanding mis-implementation in public health practice. *Am J Prev Med.* 2015;48(5):543–551. https://doi.org/10.1016/j.amepre.2014.11.015
21. Baumann AA, Cabassa LJ. Reframing implementation science to address inequities in healthcare delivery. *BMC Health Serv Res.* 2020;20(1):190. https://doi.org/10.1186/s12913-020-4975-3
22. Brownson RC, Kumanyika SK, Kreuter MW, Haire-Joshu D. Implementation science should give higher priority to health equity. *Implement Sci.* 2021;16(1):28. https://doi.org/10.1186/s13012-021-01097-0
23. Shelton RC, Chambers DA, Glasgow RE. An extension of RE-AIM to enhance sustainability: addressing dynamic context and promoting health equity over time. *Front Public Health.* 2020;8:134. https://doi.org/10.3389/fpubh.2020.00134
24. Djulbegovic B, Guyatt GH. Progress in evidence-based medicine: a quarter century on. *Lancet.* 2017;390(10092):415–423. https://doi.org/10.1016/S0140-6736(16)31592-6
25. Brownson RC, Gurney JG, Land GH. Evidence-based decision making in public health. *J Public Health Manag Pract.* 1999;5(5):86–97. https://doi.org/10.1097/00124784-199909000-00012
26. Glasziou P, Longbottom H. Evidence-based public health practice. *Aust N Z J Public Health.* 1999;23(4):436–440. https://doi.org/10.1111/j.1467-842X.1999.tb01291.x
27. Jenicek M. Epidemiology, evidence-based medicine, and evidence-based public health. *J Epidemiol.* 1997;7(4):187–197. https://doi.org/10.2188/jea.7.187
28. Brownson RC, Fielding JE, Maylahn CM. Evidence-based public health: A fundamental concept for public health practice. *Annu Rev Public Health.* 2009;30(1):175–201. https://doi.org/10.1146/annurev.publhealth.031308.100134
29. Community Preventive Services Task Force. The Community Guide. Centers for Disease Control and Prevention. 2023. Available at: https://thecommunityguide.org. Accessed February 29, 2024.

30. Cochrane. The Cochrane Collaboration. Available at: http://www.cochrane.org. Accessed August 7, 2023.
31. University of Wisconsin Population Health Institute. Using what works for health. County Health Rankings. Available at: https://www.countyhealthrankings.org/strategies-and-solutions/what-works-for-health. Accessed August 7, 2023.
32. Bor J, Cohen GH, Galea S. Population health in an era of rising income inequality: USA, 1980–2015. *Lancet.* 2017;389(10077):1475–1490. https://doi.org/10.1016/S0140-6736(17)30571-8
33. Krieger N. Enough: COVID-19, structural racism, police brutality, plutocracy, climate change—and time for health justice, democratic governance, and an equitable, sustainable future. *Am J Public Health.* 2020;110(11):1620–1623. https://doi.org/10.2105/AJPH.2020.305886
34. Kumanyika SK. Health equity is the issue we have been waiting for. *J Public Health Manag Pract.* 2016;22(suppl 1):S8–S10. https://doi.org/10.1097/PHH.0000000000000363
35. de Beaumont Foundation. Key findings of PH WINS 2014. Available at: https://debeaumont.org/phwins/2014-findings. Accessed August 5, 2023.
36. de Beaumont Foundation. 2021 Public Health Workforce Interests and Needs Survey. Available at: https://debeaumont.org/phwins/2021-findings. Accessed August 5, 2023.
37. Masters R, Anwar E, Collins B, Cookson R, Capewell S. Return on investment of public health interventions: a systematic review. *J Epidemiol Community Health.* 2017;71(8):827–834. https://doi.org/10.1136/jech-2016-208141
38. Kingdon JW. *Agendas, Alternatives, and Public Policies, Update Edition, With an Epilogue on Health Care.* Updated 2nd ed. London, England: Pearson; 2010.
39. Strassheim H, Kettunen P. When does evidence-based policy turn into policy-based evidence? Configurations, contexts and mechanisms. *Evid Policy.* 2014;10(2):259–277. https://doi.org/10.1332/174426514X13990433991320
40. Butler D, Volden C, Dynes A, Shor B. Ideology, learning, and policy diffusion: experimental evidence. *Am J Political Sci.* 2017;61(1):37–49.
41. National Center for Health Statistics. *Healthy People 2020 Overview of Health Disparities. Healthy People 2020 Final Review.* 2022. Available at: https://www.cdc.gov/nchs/healthy_people/hp2020/health-disparities.htm. Accessed February 29, 2024.
42. Arias E, Tejada-Vera B, Kochanek K, Ahmad F. Provisional life expectancy estimates for 2021. Vital Statistics Rapid Release. Hyattsville, MD: National Center for Health Statistics; August 2022.
43. Virginia Commonwealth University. Mapping life expectancy. Center on Society and Health. Available at: https://societyhealth.vcu.edu/work/the-projects/mapping-life-expectancy.html#gsc.tab=0. Accessed August 4, 2023.
44. MacKinnon NJ, Emery V, Waller J, et al. Mapping health disparities in 11 high-income nations. *JAMA Netw Open.* 2023;6(7):e2322310. https://doi.org/10.1001/jamanetworkopen.2023.22310
45. Goldberg DS. Against the very idea of the politicization of public health policy. *Am J Public Health.* 2012;102(1):44–49. https://doi.org/10.2105/AJPH.2011.300325
46. Heltzel G, Laurin K. Polarization in America: two possible futures. *Curr Opin Behav Sci.* 2020;34:179–184. https://doi.org/10.1016/j.cobeha.2020.03.008
47. Fraser T, Aldrich DP, Panagopoulos C, Hummel D, Kim D. The harmful effects of partisan polarization on health. *PNAS Nexus.* 2022;1(1):pgac011. https://doi.org/10.1093/pnasnexus/pgac011
48. Greenblatt A. Public health struggles with pandemic and politics. *Governing.* August 19, 2021. Available at: https://www.governing.com/now/public-health-struggles-with-pandemic-and-politics. Accessed February 29, 2024.
49. Ward JA, Stone EM, Mui P, Resnick B. Pandemic-related workplace violence and its impact on public health officials, March 2020–January 2021. *Am J Public Health.* 2022;112(5):736–746. https://doi.org/10.2105/AJPH.2021.306649
50. Topazian RJ, McGinty EE, Han H, et al. US adults' beliefs about harassing or threatening public health officials during the COVID-19 pandemic. *JAMA Netw Open.* 2022;5(7):e2223491. https://doi.org/10.1001/jamanetworkopen.2022.23491
51. Meier BM, Evans DP, Kavanagh MM, Keralis JM, Armas-Cardona G. Human rights in public health: deepening engagement at a critical time. *Health Hum Rights.* 2018;20(2):85–91.
52. United Nations. *Universal Declaration of Human Rights.* December 10, 1948. Available at: https://www.un.org/en/about-us/universal-declaration-of-human-rights. Accessed February 29, 2024.
53. McGowan AK, Lee MM, Meneses CM, Perkins J, Youdelman M. Civil rights laws as tools to advance health in the twenty-first century. *Annu Rev Public Health.* 2016;37(1):185–204. https://doi.org/10.1146/annurev-publhealth-032315-021926
54. Gruskin S, Loff B. Do human rights have a role in public health work? *Lancet.* 2002;360(9348):1880. https://doi.org/10.1016/S0140-6736(02)11780-6
55. Brown CL, Raza D, Pinto AD. Voting, health and interventions in healthcare settings: a scoping review. *Public Health Rev.* 2020;41(1):16. https://doi.org/10.1186/s40985-020-00133-6
56. APHA Policy Statement: Advancing health equity through protecting and promoting access to voting. Policy No. 20229. Washington, DC: American Public Health Association; November 8, 2022.
57. Jackson J, Stewart AM, Fleegler EW. Down but not defeated: clinicians can harness the power of policy for LGBTQ+ rights. *Prev Med.* 2023;167:107423. https://doi.org/10.1016/j.ypmed.2023.107423
58. Krieger N. Public health, embodied history, and social justice: looking forward. *Int J Health Serv.* 2015;45(4):587–600. https://doi.org/10.1177/0020731415595549
59. Orr JM, Leider J, Hogg-Graham R, et al. Contemporary public health finance: varied definitions, patterns, and implications. *Annu Rev Public Health.* 2023; epub ahead of print December 18, 2023. https://doi.org/10.1146/annurev-publhealth-013023-111124
60. Erwin PC, Brownson RC. The public health practitioner of the future. *Am J Public Health.* 2017;107(8):1227–1232. https://doi.org/10.2105/AJPH.2017.303823

Thirty-Six Years After the 1988 IOM *Future of Public Health*: Stop Ruminating and Start Taking Action

Angela K. McGowan, JD, MPH, Stephen Greeley, MS, Rya Griffis, MPH, and Susan L. Polan, PhD

ABOUT THE AUTHORS

Angela K. McGowan, Rya Griffis, and Susan L. Polan are with the American Public Health Association, Washington, DC. Stephen Greeley is with Shared Cause, Alexandria, VA.

See also The 1988 IOM Report, pp. 453, 461, and 467–500.

AJPH May 2024, Vol. 114, No. 5

The main goals of the Institute of Medicine's 1988 report *The Future of Public Health*[1] are laudable and still necessary today. This report recognized that the mission of public health is "fulfilling society's interest in assuring conditions in which people can be healthy."[1(p7)] To achieve this, all levels of the governmental public health field—federal, state, local, and tribal—must be engaged in addressing the defined core functions. One major concern, as the COVID-19 pandemic has demonstrated, is that 36 years later, although we have made improvements, the overarching goals of the report remain aspirational.

The COVID-19 pandemic brought into sharp focus the need for a cross-sector, multidisciplinary approach, and the American Public Health Association responded by organizing the Alliance for Disease Prevention and Response.[2] The Alliance is a collaborative initiative focusing on advancing a strong public health system for everyone and includes 80 cross-sectoral organizations. The Alliance has received support from the CDC Foundation, Kaiser Permanente, the Rockefeller Foundation, the Skoll Foundation, and the W.K. Kellogg Foundation. The Alliance's goal is to accelerate building a robust and resilient public health system that advances health and well-being for all.

After extensive study and input from the public health community and cross-sectoral and community-based partners, we believe a key next step is to launch a large cross-sectoral movement, including an action arm, the Campaign for the Public's Health, to expand active engagement and collaboration and champion advances in public health and equity. This will involve catalyzing community-level partnership, communicating a shared vision, and jointly advocating supportive policy and system building. Linchpins of these efforts are collaboration and alignment, avoiding redundancy, and identifying organizations ready to lead, champion, support, and amplify the work of others to reach shared goals.

BACKGROUND

To determine priorities for this movement and the Campaign for the Public's Health, the Alliance undertook a comprehensive and collaborative process of reviewing and summarizing more than 100 recommendations from 13 recently released reports or activities focusing on improving the public health system, including those from the Bipartisan Policy Center,[3] the Commonwealth Fund,[4] the Robert Wood Johnson Foundation,[5] CDC Foundation's Lights Camera Action series,[6] and the President's Council on Science and Technology.[7] We identified four major focus areas: (1) data and information technology; (2) law and governance; (3) social determinants of health, equity, and partnerships; and (4) the workforce. The vetting process, which involved more than 200 individuals, identified an agenda with focused priorities for the public health system. The process also identified the need for the public health community to better employ tools and tactics, including advocacy, communications, and partnerships, and to better engage communities; it also reinforced several key lessons.

KEY LESSONS

Here are the broader lessons we learned, which are part of any comprehensive campaign and which we must consider to achieve the goal of building a robust and resilient public health system that improves health for all and better learns from and supports community coalitions:

1. Stop ruminating and start taking action! Although we have seen advances over the past 36 years, we have not seen the necessary wide-scale changes identified in the 1988 report. Some things have improved: diseases are close to being eradicated or are treatable, more data are available, information is shared rapidly, and environments are cleaner. But we still face

major challenges in supporting wellness for all and preventing or responding to major threats and building trust in the public health community. We must begin to move past analysis and research to implement the critical changes outlined in these reports and advance this movement with necessary resources, partners, and authority.

2. Recognize the broader focus that is critical to improving the public's health. The social determinants of health, without necessary policy solutions or the will required to fix them, can be primary factors in exacerbating health inequities. The move from focusing on health inequities to addressing health equity has been crucial, but as a field we still need to continue to move forward and to address some of the structural barriers such as poverty, discrimination, or environmental threats that cause many inequities. The incorporation of new partners, communities, and other fields has helped us address these necessary precursors to health in many places.

3. Governmental public health is core to improving the public's health but cannot do it alone. To promote and protect health, many issues, programs, functions, and capacities must be called on from outside the public health governmental infrastructure. The pandemic showed the need for collaboration with partners, including health care workers, social service providers, businesses, schools, faith-based organizations, and community residents of all backgrounds. The institution of public health has created social movements and worked to ensure everyone has the opportunity to live their healthiest lives, but large-scale societal changes to improve well-being for everyone in every community across the nation happen through collaboration and aligned action.

4. Community must be central to this work. Improving the health of communities that are underserved and disproportionately excluded from decision-making through power sharing and active listening must become central to public health practice. Many coalitions responded to the COVID-19 pandemic, although their primary focus was on other health and social determinants of health issues affecting their communities, and they provided the opportunity for residents to advocate for themselves. Challenges include identifying funding sources for basic coalition capacity; engaging local, resident-driven coalitions; and providing them with the information and tools they need to be effective.

5. The public health field is political but not partisan. Although science and evidence are core to public health practice, during the pandemic many public health decisions were made publicly in the policy or political realm. As a result, the public health field became a political target. Our leaders and practitioners must learn to regularly engage with decision-makers and advocate for public health at all levels of government. The public health community needs to celebrate successes, learn how to explain what we do to new and nonscientific audiences, and make new partners. Having community or cross-sectoral partners elevate the value of public health would provide some credence and justification for additional funding, projects, or partnerships.

6. We must learn to play the long game. The pandemic reinforced the importance of public health and preparing for emergencies. Although the field cobbled together a response and prevented an even more dire outcome, the struggle revealed the impacts of long-term underinvestment in public health. We need to better explain prevention and the value of public health and the necessity of a trained, supported, and well-compensated workforce and strong data systems. We must ensure that officials have the authority to act to protect the public and its health and invest in preparedness to allow planning and resources to act. We must encourage political leaders and funders to look beyond the short-term nature of election cycles, crisis-driven responses, or Congressional Budget Office scoring and instead make long-term consistent investments to build the public health system of the future.

7. Collaboration and aligning efforts are key. Finally, public health is too compartmentalized and, in many places, unfocused. We need to come together and better coordinate messages, lessons, and actions to ensure progress on a common agenda. Creating a movement and the Campaign for the Public's Health are steps in that direction.

By working together with partners, the public health community must begin to take action toward the aspirational vision shared in many reports and recommendations. Hopefully, we can move forward from rhetoric, research, and reactive responses toward collective and proactive action to achieve large-scale changes in the health and well-being of all. AJPH

CORRESPONDENCE

Correspondence should be sent to Susan Polan, American Public Health Association, Public Affairs and Advocacy, 800 I St NW, Washington, DC 20001 (e-mail: susan.polan@apha.org). Reprints can be ordered at http://www.ajph.org by clicking the "Reprints" link.

PUBLICATION INFORMATION

Full Citation: McGowan AK, Greeley S, Griffis R, Polan SL. Thirty-six years after the 1988 IOM *Future of Public Health*: stop ruminating and start taking action. *Am J Public Health*. 2024;114(5): 486–488.

Acceptance Date: February 15, 2024.

DOI: https://doi.org/10.2105/AJPH.2024.307634

CONTRIBUTORS

A. K. McGowan was the primary author of the editorial. S. Greeley and R. Griffis contributed to editing the editorial. S. L. Polan provided significant input to the writing. All of the authors are and will continue to be actively involved in the conceptualization of the Alliance for Disease Prevention and Response and the Campaign for the Public's Health on which this editorial is based.

ACKNOWLEDGMENTS

This work was generously supported by the CDC Foundation (grant 1085.1) and the W.K. Kellogg Foundation (grant P-6000820-2021).

The authors wish to acknowledge the work of many partners and collaborators. This includes the Alliance for Disease Prevention and Response's Leadership Committee, colleagues from ICF International Inc., the Accelerator Convening team, the more than 200 people who participated in vetting or learning sessions or meetings, and Alliance staff, partners, and interns who provided valuable assistance, including Georges C. Benjamin, MD, Kelly Nowlin, Bradley Bauer, Megan Collins, Roman Kassaraba, Saril May, Iesha Reid, and Sara Ukani.

Note. The contents of this editorial are solely the responsibility of the authors and do not necessarily represent the official views of the funders.

CONFLICTS OF INTEREST

The authors have no conflicts of interest to disclose.

REFERENCES

1. Institute of Medicine. *The Future of Public Health*. Washington, DC: National Academies Press; 1988.
2. American Public Health Association. Alliance for Disease Prevention and Response. Available at: https://www.apha.org/About-APHA/Centers-and-Programs/Alliance-for-Disease-Prevention. Accessed September 11, 2023.
3. Armooh T, Barton T, Castillo G, et al. Public health forward: modernizing the US public health system. December 2021. Available at: https://bipartisanpolicy.org/download/?file=/wp-content/uploads/2021/12/BPC_Public-Health-Forward_R01_WEB.pdf. Accessed January 18, 2024.
4. Hamburg MA, Cohen M, DeSalvo K, et al. Meeting America's public health challenge. June 21, 2022. Available at: https://www.commonwealthfund.org/publications/fund-reports/2022/jun/meeting-americas-public-health-challenge. Accessed September 8, 2023.
5. Christopher GC, Zimmerman EB, Chandra A, Martin LT. Charting a course for an equity-centered data system: recommendations from the National Commission to Transform Public Health Data Systems. October 2021. Available at: https://www.nationalcollaborative.org/wp-content/uploads/2021/11/RWJF-Transforming-Public-Health-Data-Systems.pdf. Accessed September 8, 2023.
6. Lights, Camera, Action. The future of public health national summit series. 2021–2023. Available at: https://futureofpublichealth.org. Accessed September 11, 2023.
7. President's Council of Advisors on Science and Technology. Report to the President: supporting the US public health workforce. May 2023. Available at: https://www.whitehouse.gov/wp-content/uploads/2023/04/PCAST_Public-Health-Report_May2023.pdf. Accessed September 11, 2023.

The Influence of the 1988 and 2003 IOM *Future of Public Health* Reports on the CDC

Edward L. Baker, MD, MPH

See also The 1988 IOM Report, pp. 453, 461, and 467–500.

The landmark 1988 Institute of Medicine report *The Future of Public Health* served the public health community well by pointing to what needed to be done, fostering a sense of urgency, and offering concrete directions to be pursued.

In this article, the impact of the 1988 report, and of the subsequent 2003 report on the Centers for Disease Control and Prevention (CDC), is considered by tracing the course of the ideas that influenced the consciousness of the public health community and subsequently catalyzed concrete action. Among these ideas was that "public health is in disarray." This assessment led to an awareness that something needed to be done. Further, by stating that the public health enterprise had 3 core functions (assessment, policy development, and assurance), the 1988 report set in motion policy development to address the "disarray."

At a more fundamental level, both reports championed the need for governmental public health (particularly at the CDC) to take action to strengthen the capacity of local and state public health agencies to address a growing range of public health threats and emergencies. (*Am J Public Health*. 2024;114(5):489–494. https://doi.org/10.2105/AJPH.2024.307598)

AJPH May 2024, Vol. 114, No. 5

The landmark 1988 Institute of Medicine (IOM) report *The Future of Public Health*[1] and its subsequent 2003 report[2] influenced a range of Centers for Disease Control and Prevention (CDC) programs and perspectives. As a result, CDC programs were created to respond to the "call to action" of these seminal reports. At a fundamental level, both reports championed the need for the CDC, along with its partners, to take concerted action to strengthen the nation's public health system.

CONTEXT

The 1988 report came out during a period of seminal research and policy development focusing on building the capacity of the public health system to address a widening range of health challenges. Prior to 1988, research had revealed a high degree of variability in the range of services provided by local health agencies across the nation. To address this high level of variability, visionary leaders at that time developed a list of 10 public health practices as an initial basis for standardization of public health services at the local and state levels.[3] This listing was used by academic researchers to assess the capacity and practices of local and state health agencies, thereby providing objective evidence for the "disarray" noted in the 1988 report.

In addition, the 1990 Health Objectives for the Nation built on other initiatives to enhance public health capacity. Throughout the decades of the 1980s and 1990s, tools were developed to assist local and state health agencies in strategic planning and partnership development. The first tool was APEXPH (Assessment Protocol for Excellence in Public Health), which was then followed by a widely used capacity-building tool created by the National Association of County and City Health Officials: MAPP (Mobilizing for Action Through Planning and Partnerships: A Community Approach to Health Improvement).[4] These and other initiatives acted synergistically with the 1988 report to foster concerted action to strengthen public health agency capacity and to influence leaders to act.

Then, the 2003 report built upon the conceptual framework of the 1988 report by endorsing a range of conclusions and recommendations from the earlier report and by acknowledging the progress made over a 15-year period. The 2003 report acknowledged the progress made in creating a list of 10 Essential Public Health Services on which the CDC-led National Public Health Performance Standards were based. The 2003 report also advocated for the creation of a national system to accredit local and state governmental public health agencies.[2] Between 1988 and 2003, the use of computerized information systems exploded, with profound implications for the public health enterprise; the 2003 report acknowledged progress made to strengthen the public health information infrastructure since 1988, but noted that much more work was needed.

IMPACT ON THE CDC

Central to the 1988 report was the thesis that action at the federal level was essential to address the shortcomings in the nation's public health system. In general, the report was instrumental in advancing the concept that the CDC should commit to efforts to strengthen the nation's public health system. Accordingly, this article highlights the influence of ideas contained in the 1988 report on certain CDC programs and priorities. The process, which was catalyzed by the 1988 report, played out over the decade of the 1990s and beyond. In order for the ideas noted in the report to effect action through policies and programs, leadership was an essential ingredient.

LEADERSHIP

On March 1, 1990, Bill Roper became CDC director. I was most fortunate that I started my tenure as director of the CDC Public Health Practice Program Office on the same day in 1990. Shortly after Roper became CDC director, he articulated 3 top priorities for the CDC, one of which was "Strengthening the Public Health System."[5] Because Roper had served as a local health department director in Birmingham, Alabama and had studied the public health system as a public health graduate student at the University of Alabama at Birmingham, he was well aware of the issues cited in the 1988 report. As a result of his leadership, the wheels were set in motion for innovative action over the coming decades.

Subsequently, other CDC directors, notably David Satcher and Jeffrey Koplan, continued to support a range of efforts to strengthen the public health infrastructure and to broaden the focus (as noted in the 2003 report) to reach out to community-based organizations (under Satcher's leadership). After the terrorist attacks of September 11, 2001 and the subsequent anthrax attacks, Koplan successfully advocated for major increases in support for state and public health capacity such that the CDC fiscal year (FY) 2002 budget increased substantially—by $865 million annually—with $110 million earmarked for the Health Alert Network along with other initiatives (e.g., epidemiological capacity, lab capacity, preparedness planning, and education and training). These areas of need were identified both in the 1988 report and in the 2003 report. This increased funding continued for several years after the FY2002 funding cycle.

FROM DISARRAY TO STANDARDIZATION AND ACCREDITATION

The 1988 report took the first step along the path from "disarray" to the present system of health agency accreditation by stating that public health had 3 core functions: assessment, policy development, and assurance. Once these core functions were articulated, public health leaders began to support the concept that greater uniformity of public health services was desirable. However, these broad concepts needed further refinement to enhance policymakers' understanding of what public health does. So, a set of 10 Essential Public Health Services was created to elaborate more concretely on the IOM's list of 3 core functions.[6]

Once the 10 Essential Public Health Services were described, public health leaders used that framework to build out initiatives that were designed to move from disarray to standardization. This process, led by Paul Halverson and Bud Nicola, was based on the maxim that "what gets measured gets done," and produced a set of detailed National Public Health Performance Standards, which formed a blueprint for action. These standards provided a uniform, outcome-based model for evaluating public health programs, which was then used to guide action at the state and local levels.[7]

Flowing from the creation of these Performance Standards, accreditation of local and state health agencies constituted a further step toward addressing the "disarray" noted in the 1988 report.[7] As a further step in that process, the Exploring Accreditation Project was launched in 2005, followed by the creation of the nonprofit Public Health Accreditation Board (PHAB) in 2007.[8] This voluntary system of accrediting state and local health agencies began the accreditation process in 2011. Since that time, PHAB has continued to accredit public health departments to strengthen public health infrastructure and transform governmental public health. To date, 41 state health departments, 321 local health departments, and 6 tribal health departments have been accredited. As a result, 90% of the US population is served by an accredited health department. The vast majority (95%) of accredited health departments say accreditation stimulated quality and performance improvement, 77% say accreditation strengthened relationships with key partners, and 65% say accreditation improved the use of resources.[8]

The COVID-19 pandemic has been a significantly difficult time for many health departments. However, many accredited health departments have found accreditation to have been helpful in their preparedness for the pandemic. More than 80% of health departments indicated that, overall, accreditation has helped their response to the pandemic. Preparation for accreditation has been particularly helpful in response to the COVID-19 pandemic in the areas of preparedness plans and policies and relationships with other sectors and stakeholders.[9]

WORKFORCE DEVELOPMENT AND PUBLIC HEALTH EDUCATION

In addition to influencing the course of organizational development, the 1988 report catalyzed CDC initiatives to strengthen the public health workforce.[10] These initiatives were designed to enhance a range of technical skills as well as leadership and management skills.

Technical Skill Development

The CDC had a long history of providing training and career development for the public health workforce. However, access to CDC training was limited; as noted in the 1988 report, developing the technical skills of the workforce in core areas (e.g., immunization practices) was essential for the future of public health. To address these needs, the CDC created the Public Health Training Network in 1993, which employed innovative distance learning techniques to enhance the reach of CDC training programs under the leadership of Dennis McDowell and other pioneers. As a result, a national public health training infrastructure was created that ultimately served over 1 million health professionals with timely training related to current threats[10]. Since then, the CDC has continued to support access to training materials for the public health workforce.

Leadership and Management Development

Another important conclusion from the 1988 report was the value of formal leadership development programs. The CDC took this charge seriously and embarked on a journey to establish a more systematic approach for developing public health leaders. The first step was the creation of the national Public Health Leadership Institute (PHLI), a flagship program, which ultimately served 1000 scholars from 1992 to 2011. An evaluation of the PHLI program demonstrated that it promoted new ways of thinking and new partnerships across the public health community.[11,12]

Further, a national network of state and regional public health leadership institutes was formed that reached thousands more individuals, enhancing thought leadership nationwide. The benefits of these programs continue to be felt to this day, as those who participated continue to apply skills and perspectives gained from these development programs. In addition to these programs, many other public health leadership development programs have been created for a range of audiences and focus areas (e.g., environmental health) over subsequent years. The 2003 report[2] acknowledged the value of CDC-supported PHLIs at the national, state, and regional levels and advocated for continued support based on the success of these programs. Unfortunately, CDC support for PHLIs was abandoned in 2011 and most programs closed their doors.

Once leadership development was under way and gaining wide support, a need for a companion system for the development of management skills was acknowledged. To address that need, the Management Academy for Public Health was launched in the late 1990s, led by Janet Porter and Jim Johnson at the University of North Carolina.[13] This program, which was supported by a consortium including the Robert Wood Johnson Foundation, the Kellogg Foundation, the Health Resources and Services Administration, and the CDC, ultimately reached hundreds of frontline public health managers with core management skills training.[13] Support from the de Beaumont Foundation served to sustain and strengthen the Management Academy after the initial phase of operations.

Public Health Education

The 1988 and 2003 reports made extensive recommendations designed to strengthen the roles of schools of public health in contributing to the education and training of the public health workforce. These recommendations related both to curriculum change for students as well as short courses for existing public health workers. These recommendations set in motion discussions designed to bridge the gap between academia and the practice community that the report delineated. Programs were launched by the CDC that began to address the gaps noted in the 1988 report. These programs, led by Maureen Lichtveld and Joan Cioffi, included the creation of Centers for Public Health Preparedness at schools of public health, followed by Preparedness and Emergency Response Learning Centers and the Preparedness and Emergency Response Research Centers.[14] Unfortunately, CDC support for these academically based programs ceased despite a clear recommendation in the 2003 report[2] that these very successful programs should continue and be strengthened to further serve the needs of the public health workforce.

THE BIRTH AND GROWTH OF PUBLIC HEALTH INFORMATICS

Although the word "informatics" does not appear in the 1988 report, that report and the 2003 report highlighted the need for improving the ways in which public health agencies manage data and information. As the computer revolution was reshaping life more broadly in the early 1990s, public health was being left behind as the Internet extended into organizational and daily life. The need for improved data and information management was once again highlighted during the COVID-19 pandemic as community leaders required better information to guide policy and practice.

During the late 1980s and early 1990s, CDC pioneers began to envision a future in which data and information could be managed more effectively and efficiently. A microcomputer-based tool—Epi Info—was created by a team led by Andy Dean and his son Jeff Dean to assist epidemiologists in carrying out standard tasks in their work; this tool is still in wide use today.[15] Another innovation—CDC WONDER, created by a team led by Howard Ory—provided online access to CDC data and information needed for epidemiological research; CDC WONDER is also in current use around the world.[15]

Following the publication of the 1988 report, the CDC undertook major initiatives to enhance the information infrastructure of state and local health agencies. The first such initiative—the Information Network for Public Health Officials (INPHO), led by Dave Ross—was designed to connect health departments to the Internet (a revolutionary concept in 1992); support the use of e-mail; enhance information access, including the creation of Web sites by public health agencies; and provide a platform to support access to distance learning from the CDC over the Internet.[15] The INPHO initiative championed the concept that the public health system must move into the "information age" and adopt innovative techniques to manage and share information.

Later, the Health Alert Network was created in the late 1990s as a response to the growing concerns about bioterrorism. This initiative, managed by a team led by Patrick O'Carroll, followed the conceptual foundation established by the INPHO project and reinforced the need to act as stated in the 1988 IOM report. Ultimately, the CDC Health Alert Network initiative achieved the goal of having every local and state health department connected to the Internet with high-speed continuous connection.[16] Today, the Health Alert Network is used regularly by the CDC and state health agencies to notify the public health system regarding health threats and emergencies. The first Health Alert Network message was sent on September 11, 2001, following the terrorist attacks on the World Trade Center and the Pentagon. Most recently, Health Alert Network Message #495 (sent on June 30, 2023) addressed the threat of exposure to wildfire smoke and Message #494 notified the public health community regarding cases of domestically acquired malaria.[17]

In 2022, the CDC launched the Data Modernization Initiative as a next step in this journey. Fueled by substantial funding, the initiative is designed to continue the process set in motion by the recommendations of the 1988 and 2003 reports to improve health information systems needed to support the work of public health agencies.[18] Ultimately, this and other initiatives are designed to create a national network of "informatics savvy health departments" with the capacity and capability to manage and share public health data and information for the communities which they serve.[19]

During the years following the 2 IOM reports, efforts to unify public health information systems were challenged by the plethora of information systems designed to support categorical disease programs, As noted in the 2003 report, failure to integrate public health information systems represented a clear threat to the ability of the public health system to effectively manage information in the event of a major public health emergency by employing interoperable approaches. Recent events, including the COVID-19 pandemic, have validated the observations of the 2003 report. Hopefully, the Data Modernization Initiative now under way may address many of the shortcomings of the fragmented public health information infrastructure.

OTHER CDC-LED INITIATIVES

The momentum for public health system change that was set in motion by the 1988 report continued well beyond the initial years following publication of the report. These "downstream" initiatives included the creation of a Guide to Community Preventive Services, which has served public health for over 25 years in providing evidence-based practices for population health.[20] Further, the CDC established the Public Health Law program (led by Gene Matthews, Rick Goodman, and Tony Moulton) during this period to support the legal foundation of the public health enterprise.[21] The 2003 report[2] highlighted the need to revamp public statutes at the national and state levels and documented early work to achieve this goal. Recently, the Robert Wood Johnson Foundation led the creation of a national network of regional public health law centers, which are carrying on the work highlighted in the 2003 report.

OBSTACLES AND FUTURE CHALLENGES

The initiatives noted here focused on the need to address systemic issues within the public health system. As in any major change initiative, obstacles and resistance to change occurred and continue to this day. Perhaps the greatest source of resistance to change was attributable to the "categorical mindset" of most CDC programs. One of the major strengths of the CDC has been the expanding focus on a range of categorical disease prevention programs, which evolved from infectious disease prevention in the early years and now include prevention of chronic diseases, injuries, health issues related to environmental and occupational hazards, the opioid epidemic, and other areas. An unfortunate unintended consequence of this expansion was that many CDC programs tended to focus on their specific area of interest with little attention to the needs of the public health system more broadly. One manifestation of this mindset is the proliferation of multiple surveillance systems for each CDC-funded program that are not interoperable, leading to inefficiency at the state and local levels.[18] Hopefully, the Data Modernization Initiative will begin to address these "data silo" issues.

Despite the progress noted here, there remain many future challenges to fulfilling the recommendations and findings of the IOM reports. Continuing the progress made toward national accreditation of public health agencies is central to addressing the "disarray" noted decades ago; CDC support, with increased attention to incentives and policy innovation, is needed to foster broader implementation of the PHAB program. Improved public health information systems are central to positioning public health to respond to the next crisis and to managing the day-to-day work of the public health enterprise. Finally, enhanced advocacy skills among public health leaders will be essential to bolster support for the work of public health at the local, state, and national levels.[22]

CONCLUSION

The 1988 IOM report *The Future of Public Health* and the 2003 report *The Future of the Public's Health* lived up to their names by offering ideas that influenced the thinking of public health leaders about the future. Further, these ideas, along with other forces at work in the decades that followed, led to specific programs that fulfilled the vision that the CDC embrace the priority of strengthening the public health infrastructure.[23] These initiatives have demonstrated lasting benefits by fostering innovation and serving the needs of those who practice public health across the nation today. Those who contributed to the creation of these reports can be justifiably proud of their seminal contributions to the present public health structures and functions, with continuing efforts for an even better future of public health. AJPH

ABOUT THE AUTHOR

Edward L. Baker is with the Schools of Public Health at the University of North Carolina, Chapel Hill, and at Harvard University, Boston, MA.

CORRESPONDENCE

Correspondence should be sent to Edward Baker, 25 Vassal Lane, Cambridge, MA 02138 (e-mail: edwardlbaker@gmail.com). Reprints can be ordered at http://www.ajph.org by clicking the "Reprints" link.

PUBLICATION INFORMATION

Full Citation: Baker EL. The influence of the 1988 and 2003 IOM *Future of Public Health* reports on the CDC. *Am J Public Health*. 2024;114(5):489–494.

Acceptance Date: January 17, 2024.

DOI: https://doi.org/10.2105/AJPH.2024.307598

CONFLICTS OF INTEREST

The author has no conflicts of interest to declare.

HUMAN PARTICIPANT PROTECTION

No protocol approval was necessary because this article did not involve human participants.

REFERENCES

1. Institute of Medicine. *The Future of Public Health.* Washington, DC: National Academy Press; 1988.
2. Institute of Medicine. *The Future of the Public's Health.* Washington, DC: National Academy Press; 2003.
3. Turnock BJ, Handler A. The 10 public health practices vs the 10 public health services: a clarification. *Am J Public Health.* 1995;85(9):1295–1296. https://doi.org/10.2105/AJPH.85.9.1295-a
4. National Association of County and City Health Officials. Mobilization for Action Through Planning and Partnerships (MAPP). Available at: https://www.naccho.org/programs/public-health-infrastructure/performance-improvement/community-health-assessment/mapp. Accessed August 15, 2023.
5. Roper WL, Baker EL, Dyal WW, Nicola RM. Strengthening the public health system. *Public Health Rep.* 1992;107(6):609–615.
6. Baker EL, Melton RJ, Stange PV, et al. Health reform and the health of the public: forging community health partnerships. *JAMA.* 1994;272(16):1276–1282. https://doi.org/10.1001/jama.1994.03520160060044
7. Halverson PK, Nicola RM, Baker EL. Performance measurement and accreditation of public health organizations: a call to action. *J Public Health Manag Pract.* 1998;4(4):5–7. https://doi.org/10.1097/00124784-199807000-00004
8. Public Health Accreditation Board. Available at: https://phaboard.org. Accessed August 15, 2023.
9. Public Health Accreditation Board. The value and impact of public health department accreditation. July 2023. Available at: https://phaboard.org/wp-content/uploads/PHAB-Value-and-Impact.pdf. Accessed August 15, 2023.
10. Baker EL, Potter MA, Jones DL, et al. The public health infrastructure and our nation's health. *Annu Rev Public Health.* 2005;26(1):303–318. https://doi.org/10.1146/annurev.publhealth.26.021304.144647
11. Umble KE, Baker EL, Woltring C. An evaluation of the National Public Health Leadership Institute—1991–2006: part I. Developing individual leaders. *J Public Health Manag Pract.* 2011;17(3):202–213. https://doi.org/10.1097/PHH.0b013e3181f1e3dc
12. Umble K, Baker EL, Diehl SJ, et al. An evaluation of the National Public Health Leadership Institute—1991–2006: part II. Strengthening public health leadership networks, systems, and infrastructure. *J Public Health Manag Pract.* 2011;17(3):214–224. https://doi.org/10.1097/PHH.0b013e31820759d0
13. Porter J, Johnson J, Upshaw VM, Orton S, Deal KM, Umble K. The Management Academy for Public Health. *J Public Health Manag Pract.* 2002;8(2):66–78. https://doi.org/10.1097/00124784-200203000-00009
14. Lichtveld M, Cioffi JP. Public health workforce development: progress, challenges and opportunities. *J Public Health Manag Pract.* 2003;9(6):443–450. https://doi.org/10.1097/00124784-200311000-00003
15. Ross DA, Baker EL. A brief history of public health informatics—lessons for leaders and a look into the future. *J Public Health Manag Pract.* 2023;29(1):101–104. https://doi.org/10.1097/PHH.0000000000001672
16. Baker EL, Porter J. The Health Alert Network: partnerships, politics and preparedness. *J Public Health Manag Pract.* 2005;11(6):574–576. https://doi.org/10.1097/00124784-200511000-00017
17. Centers for Disease Control and Prevention. Health Alert Network. Available at: https://emergency.cdc.gov/han/index.asp. Accessed August 15, 2023.
18. Singletary V, Richards CL, Ross DA, O'Carroll P, Baker EL. Modernizing our nation's public health information system: toward an integrated approach. *J Public Health Manag Pract.* 2021;27(5):521–525. https://doi.org/10.1097/PHH.0000000000001400
19. LaVenture M, Brand B, Ross DA, Baker EL. Building an informatics-savvy health department: part I, vision and core strategies. *J Public Health Manag Pract.* 2014;20(6):667–669. https://doi.org/10.1097/PHH.0000000000000149
20. Community Preventive Services Task Force. The Community Guide. Available at: https://www.thecommunityguide.org. Accessed August 15, 2023.
21. Centers for Disease Control and Prevention. Public Health Law Program. Available at: https://www.cdc.gov/phlp/index.html. Accessed August 15, 2023.
22. Hearne SA, Jernigan DH, Frey M, Matthews GW, Baker EL. Strengthening advocacy skills for public health leaders. *J Public Health Manag Pract.* 2023;29(6):950–952. https://doi.org/10.1097/PHH.0000000000001827
23. Baker EL, Koplan JP. Strengthening the nation's public health infrastructure: historic challenge, unprecedented opportunity. *Health Affairs (Millwood).* 2002;21(6):15–27. https://doi.org/10.1377/hlthaff.21.6.15

Revisiting the IOM Reports and Envisioning a Promising Future for Public Health

Alina B. Baciu, PhD, MPH, and Rose Marie Martinez, ScD

See also The 1988 IOM Report, pp. 453, 461, and 467–500.

Two public health reports from the National Academies of Sciences, Engineering, and Medicine published in 1988 and 2003 by the Institute of Medicine continue to resonate.

The COVID-19 pandemic highlighted the need for a robust and adequately funded public health system that has political and public support as well as strong connections to health care and other sectors. However, a spate of recent assessments of the nation's public health infrastructure shows continuing gaps in funding, workforce, capacity, and other dimensions.

There are reasons for optimism and opportunities for progress in public health in the third decade of the 21st century. There is great promise in cross-sector partnerships and in embracing the "public" in public health by building power with communities in health improvement efforts and in decision-making. (*Am J Public Health*. 2024;114(5):495–500. https://doi.org/10.2105/AJPH.2024.307584)

AJPH May 2024, Vol. 114, No. 5

In 1988, *The Future of Public Health* (*FPH*) was published by the Institute of Medicine (IOM) at a time characterized by concerns about HIV/AIDS, rising infant mortality, outbreaks of measles, and questions about the role of government in the lives of US residents.[1] In 2003, IOM published *The Future of the Public's Health in the 21st Century* (*FPH21*) to consider progress made and changes needed to further the mission of public health in the new century. The context was similarly challenging in the aftermath of the 9/11 attacks.

Thirty-five and 20 years later, respectively, only some things have changed. The reports' key messages still resonate: public health is in disarray, there is insufficient and sporadic funding to support public health functions, more and better partnerships with other sectors and organizations are needed, and public and policymaker awareness and support are lacking. Today, the nation again finds itself at a moment for soul searching about the role of public health in society.

CHALLENGES OUTLINED IN *FPH* AND *FPH21*

FPH recommended that public health agencies

> seek stronger relationships and common cause with other professional and citizen groups pursuing interests with health implications, including voluntary health organizations, groups concerned with improving social services or the environment, and groups concerned with economic development.[1(p417)]

FPH21 built on the 1988 definition of public health (i.e., "what we, as a society, do collectively to assure the conditions in which people can be healthy"[1[p1]]) as a shared and whole-of-society undertaking.

FPH outlined core functions of public health: assessment, policy development, and assurance. It also described responsibilities for each level of government along with enabling steps (statutory, structural and organizational, and capacity building) and discussed workforce education and training needs. The report noted 2 factors that shaped how public health problems were solved: the contributions of scientific and technical knowledge and the tenor of public values and popular opinion. Much has changed in how and what information is shared and accessed by the public—with far-reaching effects on their view of public health efforts and services, their trust in government, and their perception of threats to health.

Several challenges described in *FPH* still affect US public health:

- Public and political views of the role of government as they inform considerations about the scope of government public health (i.e., narrow vs expansive);
- Inadequate and unstable funding;
- Lack of investment in public health research;
- Insufficient collaboration between and across relevant sectors, beginning with the public health–health care relationship, including in information sharing and resource allocation; and
- Inability to navigate the politicization of public health issues.

The COVID-19 pandemic demonstrated the potential of effective public health infrastructure as some state and local public health agencies, along with private-sector partners, innovated and achieved some wins in safeguarding the public's health. These include the stay-at-home orders that flattened the curve of hospitalizations in the early months of the pandemic, the rapid development and production of vaccines, and the eventual wide availability of antigen tests. However, the crisis also laid bare the continuing gaps in the public health infrastructure and funding and in the prerequisites for equitable health and well-being, such as housing, workforce protections, and economic stability, along with a lack of robust cross-sector partnerships and limited engagement with communities on decision-making.

In explaining the need for multisector action, *FPH21* noted, "Government cannot assure population health alone; other sectors and parties have an interest and a civic role to help create the conditions that make health possible."[2(p22)] The report also asserted that the nation's investments and policies accord a higher value to individual-based rather than population health approaches and to biomedical over prevention research. It identified the following shortcomings and gaps in the US public health infrastructure:

> vulnerable and outdated health information systems and technologies, an insufficient and inadequately trained public health workforce, antiquated laboratory capacity, a lack of real-time surveillance and epidemiological systems, ineffective and fragmented communications networks, incomplete domestic preparedness and emergency response capabilities.[2(p3)]

To address these challenges, the authoring committee recommended more flexible and adequate funding for public health; expanding federal funding for prevention and population- and community-based research; implementing strategies for engaging other sectors, such as business and the media, and for supporting community-led efforts to improve community health; and strengthening public health communication to demonstrate value and accountability to the public.

The time line in Table 1 lists some of the milestones that illustrate the juxtaposition of public health crises with fluctuations in public health funding (increases, followed by cuts) over the past 2 decades. Overall, the budget of the Centers for Disease Control and Prevention (CDC) fell by 2% between 2012 and 2021,[9] and public health spending stayed flat or decreased over the first 2 decades of the 21st century.[17]

BEYOND *FPH* AND *FPH21*

Between 2021 and 2023, several reports on the US public health infrastructure have been released that contain recommendations and messages that echo those of the decades-old IOM reports, especially those related to funding shortfalls and infrastructure gaps. The Bipartisan Policy Center published *Public Health Forward: Modernizing the US Public Health System*, which outlined a vision of a healthier nation (by 2026) with a public health system supported by "sufficient, predictable, and flexible public health funding"[15]; a modern, interoperable, and secure public health information system; a diverse and well-equipped workforce; modernized laws and policies; and partnerships and community engagement.

The CDC Foundation's Lights, Camera, Action 4-part summit series held in collaboration with other public health organizations explored the following dimensions of the public health system: data infrastructure, workforce, funding, and partnerships. The summit series offered fresh perspectives and calls to action that reflect contemporary concerns, evidence, and practices. These include acknowledging and repairing historical harms; democratizing data collection and sharing for narrative building that advances racial justice and health equity; engaging community members in budgeting to develop trust, share power, and build equity; addressing structural racism in public health; and shifting power dynamics.

The Commonwealth Fund Commission report *Meeting America's Public Health Challenge* outlined an expansive vision of the public health system and

TABLE 1— Time Line of Select Public Health Milestones

Year	Milestone
2001	9/11 terrorist attacks; anthrax attacks
2002–2003	Increase in total public health funding as part of emergency preparedness[3]
2005–2006	National pandemic influenza plans
2008	The Great Recession
2009	Increase in total public health funding (American Recovery and Reinvestment Act)[4]
2009–2010	H1N1 pandemic; $1.4 billion from CDC public health emergency response to support state and local public health agencies[5]
2010	Affordable Care Act provision for the prevention fund authorizes $18.75 billion in funding, intended to start at $0.5 billion/year and increase to $2 billion/year by 2015; Congress redirects funds to nonpublic health programs, decreasing the amount of funding available[6–8]
2010	The second wave of the opioid epidemic with a rapid increase in heroin-related overdose deaths (first wave in 1990s, natural and semisynthetic opioids and methadone)[7]
2012	Prevention fund cut for Medicare physician payments[9]
2013	The third wave of the opioid epidemic, with increased overdose deaths from synthetic opioids, especially illicitly produced fentanyl[7]
2014–2016	Cases of Ebola are treated in the United States[10]
2014–2016	First cases of Zika in the Americas[11]; the HHS struggles to identify resources[12]
2016	Prevention fund cut for the 21st Century Cures Act[9]
2016	The HHS articulates Public Health 3.0—denoting a new era of cross-sector collaboration for collective action (with public health agencies as "chief health strategist") and a focus on improving the social determinants of health
2018	Prevention fund cut for short-term extension of Children's Health Insurance Plan[3]
2018	The CDC budget increases $1.079 billion, including $350 million to support the opioid pandemic response[13]
2019	The fourth wave of the opioid epidemic; federal appropriations increase from $2.1 billion to $6.1 billion between 2017 and 2020[14]
2020	COVID-19 pandemic declared on March 11, 2020
2020–2021	Congress allocates $305.6 billion through 5 COVID-19 relief bills ($15.3 billion to CDC)[15]
2023	CDC faces $1.5 billion in budget cuts[16]

Note. CDC = Centers for Disease Control and Prevention; HHS = US Department of Health and Human Services; prevention fund = prevention and public health fund.

workforce.[18] This report called for mandatory, sustained funding and strategies to strengthen infrastructure so that all communities can be provided with foundational public health capabilities.[18] The report also called for creating an undersecretary of public health to provide leadership and coordination in the US Department of Health and Human Services, for adequate public health funding (supporting all aspects of the infrastructure), and for pairing funding with accountability at each level of government. Additionally, it called on all levels of government to build connections between public health and health care for both day-to-day collaboration and emergency preparedness and to involve community partners in decision-making.

These recent reports underscore long-standing problems but also reiterate the importance of partnerships and of a focus on advancing health equity, including through declarations of racism as a public health crisis.[19] This reflects shifts in the field that were merely glimpsed in *FPH* and *FPH21*. Next, we discuss promising developments and innovations in cross-sector partnerships and the role of communities in improving health, equity, and well-being.

On Cross-Sector Partnerships

There are many frameworks for and instances of effective partnerships of public health with health care and with other sectors. Some may be found in communities where hospitals, public health departments, and social sector organizations have been collaborating to conduct community health needs assessments and community health improvement planning (as called for in the Affordable Care Act and related Internal Revenue Service regulations).[20] Examples include those showcased by the Funders Forum on Accountable Health and by Communities Joined in Action.[21] There are also cross-sector partnerships with government agencies in transportation, housing, and other domains[22] and cross-sector partnerships across multiple public and private-sector organizations, such as those nurtured by the multifunder BUILD Health Challenge.[23]

But the capacity of public health agencies to build and sustain lasting partnerships across sectors remains variable and depends on idiosyncratic leaders—rather than on robust institutionalized processes—as well as funding and capacity. Often, only large, well-equipped public health agencies can build sustained relationships with community and regional partners.[24] However, examples, toolkits, and guidance on effective cross-sector collaboration are more available than ever and could assist smaller or less well-resourced public health agencies.[25]

Partnerships between public- and private-sector public health entities remain an area of enormous promise for many reasons, including better communication, greater visibility, and greater trust in and growing a constituency for public health. For example, the public health–business relationship has been discussed in a US surgeon general's report on community health and economic prosperity (https://bit.ly/3TaLshw) and a de Beaumont Foundation and Johns Hopkins University Bloomberg School of Public Health guide on alignment between business and public health leaders (https://debeaumont.org/businesspublichealth).

Several funders launched the Health Action Alliance to bring leaders in public health and business together with communication experts to help employers navigate evolving health challenges, advance health equity, and prepare for future health emergencies.[26] The COVID-19 pandemic highlighted the relationship between health and economic well-being. Despite the fog of mis- and disinformation about the virus and the vaccine, employers understood that lowering infection rates was beneficial to their business: some collaborated with public health agencies to enact policies that protected workers' health.[27]

On Community, Power, and Democracy

FPH stated, "Many public health professionals who talked with us seemed to regard politics as a contaminant of an ideally rational decision-making process rather than as an essential element of democratic governance."[1(p5)] The committee observed "little evidence of constituency building, citizen participation, or continuing (as opposed to crisis-driven) communications with elected officials or with the community at large."[1(p5)] *FPH21* asserted:

> Theories of democracy demonstrate that the public's health is an important collective good because public funds are expended to benefit all or most of the population. The public's health can be supported only through collective action, not through individual endeavor.[2(p22)]

Researchers and decision-makers acknowledge the relationship between health and democracy. In 2020, a National Academies of Sciences, Engineering, and Medicine (NASEM) report recommended, based on evidence of the relationship between health and civic engagement, that voting participation be considered for inclusion among the leading health indicators in Healthy People 2030.[28] In 2023, voting participation was added to Healthy People 2030 as a core objective.[29] The American Medical Association and the American Public Health Association recently developed and adopted policy statements recognizing voting as a social determinant of health.[30,31] In 2021, Healthy Democracy Healthy People launched the Health and Democracy Index, a Web-based tool that overlays 12 health indicators on state maps of the Cost of Voting Index (i.e., a metric of the restrictiveness of voting policies in each state; https://democracyindex.hdhp.us).

A growing number of health care organizations and providers participate in the work of Vot-ER, a national nonprofit and nonpartisan organization that works to integrate civic engagement into health care (https://vot-er.org). The nexus of civic engagement and health has also been highlighted in the NASEM report *Federal Policy to Advance Racial, Ethnic, and Tribal Health Equity*.[32] This report discusses evidence for the relationship of health and well-being with feelings of efficacy and belonging and with civic engagement. To better support states, localities, tribes, territories, and communities, the committee asserted, federal agencies should "prioritize, value, and incorporate community voice in the work of government."[32(p12)]

The evolution of community partnerships shows a maturation of the public health view of community members: service recipients, authentic partners in improving health and health equity, co-researchers, decision-makers, and leaders. Examples of such partnerships include the 24 communities that implemented the Community of Solutions Framework From 100 Million Healthier Lives' SCALE initiative, supported by the Robert Wood Johnson Foundation (RWJF),[33] the power-building work of the 14 communities in the Building Healthy Communities initiative supported by the California Endowment,[34] and the 9 community-based and cross-sector partnerships highlighted in the NASEM report *Communities in Action: Pathways to Health Equity*.[35]

There are many examples of public health collaboration with community power-building organizations that elevate the voices and expertise of community members to influence the policy agenda and change inequitable conditions for health and well-being.[36] The Health Improvement Partnership of Cuyahoga County, Ohio, is co-led by community and public health leaders working to address inequities in health and in opportunities to live long, healthy lives (https://bit.ly/3uSgoen). In Santa Barbara, California, local grassroots organizations partner with the county health department to protect farmworker health.[37] Aspects of the work of power building and its relationship with health equity have been examined by Lead Local, an effort supported by RWJF (https://www.lead-local.org). A key finding is that community members "can hold community power organizations, academics, and policymakers accountable to the community" and "push against institutional tendencies to pursue incremental change rather than transformational change."[38(p4)]

CONCLUSIONS

In 2000, the CDC published a list of the 10 greatest public health achievements of the 20th century. The list includes vaccination, control of infectious diseases, healthier mothers and babies, and family planning. As vaccine and other health disinformation is propagated on social media, and as the public dialogue refracted by the news media appears more strident and polarized on topics that include science, health, and medicine, the nation may be losing ground on these historic achievements.

How can the United States strengthen its public health infrastructure when there is an ongoing debate about the role of government in people's lives, other funding focuses take precedence, the public conflates health and health care, and decision-makers react to social problems (e.g., violence, homelessness) instead of proactively and preventively addressing vital conditions[39] for health and well-being (e.g., quality early childhood education, humane housing)? The Federal Plan for Equitable Long-Term Recovery and Resilience, an initiative begun in 2020 during the early part of the pandemic, seems to point the way forward through interagency and cross-sector efforts and through public–private and community partnerships.[39]

Governmental public health agencies must build and sustain cross-sector partnerships and put the public back in public health[40] through greater transparency and accountability and by sharing power and decision-making with the people who experience health and social inequities. Workforce development and resources, unrestricted funding, and technical assistance will be needed to develop and sustain capabilities for partnership across sectors and with communities. The ravages of the pandemic, the unfolding climate emergency, and other threats underscore the messages of *FPH* and *FPH21*: the public health system and the nation's social, economic, and democratic well-being are linked. AJPH

ABOUT THE AUTHORS

Alina B. Baciu and Rose Marie Martinez are with the Health and Medicine Division, National Academies of Sciences, Engineering, and Medicine, Washington, DC.

Note. The authors are solely responsible for the content of this paper, which does not necessarily represent the views of the National Academies of Sciences, Engineering, and Medicine.

CORRESPONDENCE

Correspondence should be sent to Alina B. Baciu, Senior Program Officer, Institute of Medicine, Board on Population Health and Public Health Practice, 500 Fifth St NW, Washington, DC 20001 (e-mail: abaciu@nas.edu). Reprints can be ordered at http://www.ajph.org by clicking the "Reprints" link.

PUBLICATION INFORMATION

Full Citation: Baciu AB, Martinez RM. Revisiting the IOM reports and envisioning a promising future for public health. *Am J Public Health*. 2024;114(5): 495–500.

Acceptance Date: January 8, 2024.

DOI: https://doi.org/10.2105/AJPH.2024.307584

CONTRIBUTORS

Alina B. Baciu and Rose Marie Martinez conceptualized and wrote the article.

CONFLICTS OF INTEREST

The authors have no conflicts of interest to declare.

HUMAN PARTICIPANT PROTECTION

No protocol approval was necessary because no human participants were involved in this work.

REFERENCES

1. Institute of Medicine. *The Future of Public Health*. Washington, DC: National Academies Press; 1988.
2. Institute of Medicine. *The Future of the Public's Health in the 21st Century*. Washington, DC: National Academies Press; 2003. https://doi.org/10.17226/10548
3. Himmelstein DU, Woolhandler S. Public health's falling share of US health spending. *Am J Public Health*. 2016;106(1):56–57. https://doi.org/10.2105/AJPH.2015.302908
4. American Public Health Association. *Prevention and Public Health Fund: Dedicated to Improving our Nation's Public Health. Advocacy Fact Sheet*. Available at: https://www.apha.org/-/media/files/pdf/factsheets/200129_pphf_factsheet.ashx. Accessed December 26, 2023.

5. Centers for Disease Control and Prevention. Public Health Emergency Response (PHER) Grant (2009-2010) for H1N1 Influenza Pandemic. Available at: https://www.cdc.gov/orr/readiness/funding_previous/funding-h1n1.htm. Accessed December 26, 2023.
6. Trust for America's Health. *The Impact of Chronic Underfunding on America's Public Health System: Trends, Risks, and Recommendations, 2022.* Available at: https://www.tfah.org/wp-content/uploads/2022/07/2022PublicHealthFundingFINAL.pdf. Accessed December 26, 2023.
7. Centers for Disease Control and Prevention. Data Analysis and Resources. 2023. Available at: https://www.cdc.gov/opioids/data/analysis-resources.html#anchor_overdose_waves. Accessed December 26, 2023.
8. Trust for America's Health. *The Impact of Chronic Underfunding on America's Public Health System: Trends, Risks, and Recommendations, 2020.* Available at: https://www.tfah.org/report-details/publichealthfunding2020. Accessed December 23, 2023.
9. Trust for America's Health. *The Impact of Chronic Underfunding on America's Public Health System: Trends, Risks, and Recommendations, 2021.* May 2021. Available at: https://www.tfah.org/wp-content/uploads/2021/05/2021_PHFunding_Fnl.pdf. Accessed December 26, 2023.
10. Chevalier MS, Chung W, Smith J, et al. Ebola virus disease cluster in the United States–Dallas County, Texas, 2014. *MMWR Morb Mortal Wkly Rep.* 2014;63(46):1087-1088. https://www.cdc.gov/mmwr/preview/mmwrhtml/mm63e1114a5.htm
11. Pan American Health Organization. Timeline - Emergence of the Zika virus in the Americas. Available at: https://www.paho.org/en/timeline-emergence-zika-virus-americas. Accessed December 23, 2023.
12. Government Accountability Office. Public Health Preparedness: HHS Reserve Funding for Emergencies. 2023. Available at: https://www.gao.gov/products/gao-23-106102. Accessed December 23, 2023.
13. Trust for America's Health. *The Impact of Chronic Underfunding on America's Public Health System: Trends, Risks, and Recommendations, 2019.* Available at: https://www.tfah.org/wp-content/uploads/2020/03/TFAH_2019_PublicHealthFunding_07.pdf. Accessed December 23, 2023.
14. Congressional Budget Office. *The Opioid Crisis and Recent Federal Policy Responses. September 2022.* Available at: https://www.cbo.gov/system/files/2022-09/58221-opioid-crisis.pdf. Accessed December 23, 2023.
15. Bipartisan Policy Center. *Public Health Forward: Modernizing the US Public Health System. 2021.* Available at https://bipartisanpolicy.org/download/?file=/wp-content/uploads/2021/12/BPC_Public-Health-Forward_R01_WEB.pdf. Accessed December 26, 2023.
16. Brozak S, Marfuggi R. The CDC faces $1.5 billion in budget cuts. Layoffs will almost certainly follow. *STAT News.* August 16, 2023. Available at: https://www.statnews.com/2023/08/16/cdc-budget-cuts-staffing-layoffs. Accessed December 26, 2023.
17. Alfonso YN, Leider JP, Resnick B, McCullough JM, Bishai D. US public health neglected: flat or declining spending left states ill equipped to respond to COVID-19. *Health Aff (Millwood).* 2021;40(4):664–671. https://doi.org/10.1377/hlthaff.2020.01084
18. Commonwealth Fund. *Meeting America's Public Health Challenge.* June 21, 2022. Available at: https://www.commonwealthfund.org/publications/fund-reports/2022/jun/meeting-americas-public-health-challenge. Accessed December 26, 2023.
19. Lights, Camera, Action. *Achieving a Diverse and Effective Public Health Workforce.* 2021. Available at: https://futureofpublichealth.org/wp-content/uploads/2022/02/LCA-Summit-1_Workforce_-Summary-Report_02.07.2022.pdf. Accessed December 26, 2023.
20. Pennel CL, Burdine JN, Prochaska JD, McLeroy KR. Common and critical components among community health assessment and community health improvement planning models. *J Public Health Manag Pract.* 2017;23(suppl 4):S14–S21. https://doi.org/10.1097/PHH.0000000000000588
21. Barnett K, Gardner E, Moore Q. *Critical Factors in Cross-Sector Health Partnerships: Charting a More Promising Future.* February 2021. Available at https://www.cjaonline.net/wp-content/uploads/2021/06/Critical-Factors-in-Cross-Sector-Health-Partnerships-Charting-a-More-Promising-Future-February-2021.pdf. Accessed December 23, 2023.
22. Association of State and Territorial Health Officials. *Initiating Cross-Sector Partnerships to Advance Population Health.* November 2021. Available at: https://www.astho.org/globalassets/report/initiating-cross-sector-partnerships-to-advance-population-health.pdf. Accessed December 26, 2023.
23. ChangeLab Solutions. *BUILDing Cross-Sector Partnerships for Health.* 2022. Available at: https://www.changelabsolutions.org/story/building-cross-sector-partnerships-health. Accessed December 26, 2023.
24. Grant AK. Patterns of cross-sector collaboration in local health departments: a cluster analysis. *Health Promot Pract.* 2022;23(1):128–136. https://doi.org/10.1177/1524839920972982
25. Georgia Health Policy Center. Aligning systems for health: health care + public health + social services. Available at: https://measuringaligning.org. Accessed December 23, 2023.
26. de Beaumont Foundation. Business & public health: working together for more prosperous communities. Available at: https://debeaumont.org/businesspublichealth. Accessed December 23, 2023.
27. Hymel P, Kassler W, Pawlecki JB. It's time to make public health a priority for business. *Fortune.* March 27, 2021. Available at: https://fortune.com/2021/03/27/business-corporate-public-health-covid. Accessed December 23, 2026.
28. National Academies of Sciences, Engineering, and Medicine. *Leading Health Indicators 2030: Advancing Health, Equity, and Well-Being.* Washington, DC: National Academies Press; 2020. https://doi.org/10.17226/25682
29. US Department of Health and Human Services. Healthy People 2030: increase the proportion of the voting-age citizens who vote—SDOH 07. Available at: https://health.gov/healthypeople/objectives-and-data/browse-objectives/social-and-community-context/increase-proportion-voting-age-citizens-who-vote-sdoh-07. Accessed December 23, 2023.
30. American Public Health Association. Advancing health equity through protecting and promoting access to voting. Policy No. 20229. November 8, 2022. Available at: https://www.apha.org/Policies-and-Advocacy/Public-Health-Policy-Statements/Policy-Database/2023/01/18/Access-to-Voting. Accessed December 23, 2023.
31. American Medical Association. Support for safe and equitable access to voting H-440.805. 2022. Available at: https://policysearch.ama-assn.org/policyfinder/detail/voting?uri=%2FAMADoc%2FHOD.xml-h-440.805.xml. Accessed December 26, 2023.
32. National Academies of Sciences, Engineering, and Medicine. *Federal Policy to Advance Racial, Ethnic, and Tribal Equity.* Washington, DC: National Academies Press; 2023.
33. Community Commons. Overview of SCALE and a community of solutions. 2017. Available at: https://www.communitycommons.org/entities/b00d5dd7-50b6-4bfd-bfb2-ae0c5219b508. Accessed December 26, 2023.
34. California Endowment. *Building Healthy Communities: A Decade in Review.* November 2020. Available at: https://www.calendow.org/app/uploads/2021/04/The_California_Endowment_Decade_In_Review_2010_2020_Executive_Report.pdf. Accessed December 23, 2023.
35. National Academies of Sciences, Engineering, and Medicine. *Communities in Action: Pathways to Health Equity.* Washington, DC: National Academies Press; 2017.
36. Heller JC, Little OM, Faust V, et al. Theory in action: public health and community power building for health equity. *J Public Health Manag Pract.* 2023;29(1):33–38. https://doi.org/10.1097/PHH.0000000000001681
37. Gaydos M, Do-Reynoso V, Williams M, Davalos H, López AJ. Power-building partnerships for health: lessons from Santa Barbara about building power to protect farmworker health and advance health equity. *J Public Health Manag Pract.* 2022;28(4 suppl 4):S166–S170. https://doi.org/10.1097/PHH.0000000000001485
38. Pastor M, Speer P, Gupta J, Han H, Ito J. Community power and health equity: closing the gap between scholarship and practice. *NAM Perspectives.* Discussion Paper, National Academy of Medicine. Washington, DC. https://doi.org/10.31478/202206c
39. US Department of Health and Human Services. *Federal Plan for Equitable Long-Term Recovery and Resilience for Social, Behavioral, and Community Health.* January 20, 2022. Available at: https://health.gov/sites/default/files/2022-04/ELTRR-Report_220127a_ColorCorrected_2.pdf. Accessed December 26, 2023.
40. Chokshi DA. Here's how CDC can put the "public" back in public health. *Scientific American.* June 30, 2023. Available at: https://www.scientificamerican.com/article/heres-how-cdc-can-put-the-public-back-in-public-health. Accessed December 26, 2023.

Per- and Polyfluoroalkyl Substance Exposure Risks in US Carceral Facilities, 2022

Lindsay Poirier, PhD, Derrick Salvatore, BS, Phil Brown, PhD, Alissa Cordner, PhD, Kira Mok, BA, and Nicholas Shapiro, DPhil

Objectives. To assess the US incarcerated population's risk of exposure to per- and polyfluoroalkyl substances (PFASs).

Methods. We assessed how many of the 6118 US carceral facilities were located in the same hydrologic unit code watershed boundaries as known or likely locations of PFAS contamination. We conducted geospatial analyses on data aggregated from Environmental Protection Agency databases and a PFAS site tracker in 2022 to model the hydrologically feasible known and presumptive PFAS contamination sites for nearly 2 million incarcerated people.

Results. Findings indicate that 5% (~310) of US carceral facilities have at least 1 known source of PFAS contamination in the same watershed boundary and that it is at a higher elevation than the facility; also 47% (~2285) have at least 1 presumptive source. A minimum of 990 000 people are incarcerated in these facilities, including at least 12 800 juveniles. Exposure risks faced by incarcerated youths are disproportionately underassessed.

Conclusions. The long-term impacts from potential exposures to PFAS are preventable and exacerbate health inequities among incarcerated populations. Widespread public attention to PFASs can be parlayed into broader environmental monitoring for imprisoned people. (*Am J Public Health*. 2024;114(5):501–510. https://doi.org/10.2105/AJPH.2024.307571)

AJPH May 2024, Vol. 114, No. 5

In recent decades, significant concerns have emerged about exposure to and associated health effects from per- and polyfluoroalkyl substances (PFASs). These substances, which are commonly referred to as "forever chemicals" because of their extreme environmental persistence, are among the highest priority emerging environmental health risks.[1] PFASs are the subject of major federal regulations, hundreds of state and federal legislative bills, major advocacy campaigns, interdisciplinary research initiatives, and multibillion-dollar lawsuit settlements.[1–4] Yet, because of protracted corporate secrecy, the difficulty and expense of testing, and slow governmental oversight, little is known about the health equity dimensions of PFAS exposures. The environmental conditions of carceral facilities are similarly difficult to research despite longstanding concerns about the environmental health of incarcerated populations owing to reduced exposure mitigation agency, health vulnerability, and racial inequity.[5–7] Connecting these critical issues, we assessed whether and how incarcerated people might be exposed to PFASs through drinking water, which is the most studied and regulated route of exposure for this family of chemicals.[1]

PFAS chemicals are a broad class of at least 12 000 chemicals. Sources of PFAS emissions to the environment include industrial emissions to water, air, or soil; use of fluorinated firefighting foams for training, testing, and fire response; application of contaminated sludge to agricultural lands; effluent discharges from wastewater treatment plants; emissions from incinerators or landfills handling PFAS-contaminated waste; and consumer uses.[8] Exposure to PFASs is associated with reproductive and developmental effects, multiple cancers, liver effects, and hormone disruption, and it is a key interest for state and federal regulators.[9] PFASs are particularly a concern for drinking water exposures, with an estimated 200 million US residents receiving PFAS-contaminated drinking water.[10] In March 2023, the US Environmental Protection Agency (EPA) proposed maximum contaminant levels for 6 PFAS, including health-based maximum contaminant-level goals for 2 PFASs at zero parts per trillion, indicating the toxicity of this chemical class at extremely low concentration.[11]

Despite research documenting PFASs' extreme persistence and ubiquitous exposure, the degree of potential exposure for the highly vulnerable incarcerated population remains unknown. The United States, which bears the highest total and per capita number of incarcerated people in the world, was home to almost 2 million people detained in prisons, jails, detention centers, and other carceral facilities,[12] with some 8.7 million people cycling through the nation's jails in 2022.[13] These populations are disproportionately Black, Latinx, Indigenous, low-income, and LGBTQ+ (lesbian, gay, bisexual, transgender/-sexual, queer or questioning, and all subsects), making the United States' exceedingly large number of carceral institutions an important window into how the justice system advances public health inequities.[6]

Incarceration—a key institution of structural racism in the United States—is also a major driver of morbidity and mortality in the United States,[5,7,14] so that 1 year of incarceration is estimated to reduce life expectancy by 2 years.[15] Both the physical health and mental health consequences of incarceration complicate employment and financial stability and are associated with reincarceration.[16] Furthermore, a study estimates that without the rise in incarceration from the 1980s to the mid-2000s, the life expectancy at birth in the United States would have increased 51% more than it did during that time.[7]

Juvenile detention is also associated with worse physical health later in life.[17] In 2019, 36 479 youths were detained or committed to a juvenile facility, and an estimated 2900 people younger than 18 years were serving time in jail.[13] Incarcerated youths are disproportionately adolescents of color, with Black youths more than 4 times as likely to be held in a juvenile facility as White youths.[18] Overrepresentation of lesbian, gay, and bisexual people in juvenile detention is driven by female lesbian, gay, and bisexual youths' detention, which is more than 3 times larger than the corresponding free population. Underlying the intersectionality of health issues facing this population, 85% of incarcerated lesbian, gay, bisexual, transgender, and gender-nonconforming incarcerated youths are people of color.[18] Between 70% and 95% of detained youth offenders have at least 1 psychiatric diagnosis,[19] yet juvenile detention and mental health services are often poorly integrated into detention facilities.

Although some mechanisms leading to health disparities for incarcerated populations, such as infectious disease, are well documented,[20] little research exists on the role of environmental contaminants. We contribute to understanding the potential environmental tributaries of the negative public health outcomes advanced by incarceration. A few studies illuminate a range of exposure routes. Toxic air releases near state prisons were found to be significantly elevated in the eastern Midwest, the Mountain region, and the Pacific region.[21] Incarcerated populations are vulnerable to heat-related mortality,[22] and EPA inspectors found a 100% violation rate across multiple hazardous waste regulations in the only known multistate prison inspection campaign.[23]

Incarcerated populations face particularly acute risks from contaminated drinking water for several reasons. First, unlike most conventional residential housing, carceral facilities can be zoned and built in industrialized areas, potentially increasing proximity to industrial exposures.[6] Second, incarcerated individuals have restricted exposure mitigation options if facilities' water becomes contaminated because of their limited or completely absent access to alternative drinking water sources or water treatment devices. Finally, because of the structural marginalization of criminalized populations, incarcerated populations have elevated chronic disease burdens that can increase an individual's risk of illness and death when facing environmental exposures.[24]

We are aware of no national studies on the drinking water quality of carceral facilities and just 2 articles on regional or subregional carceral drinking water. One study found that the water systems of carceral facilities in the US Southwest were disproportionately affected by regional exposures to arsenic.[25] Another, smaller-scale study found that a prison in California's Central Valley received drinking water violations for arsenic exceeding maximum contaminant levels for 7 years, demonstrating clear violations of the human right to water, given the health impacts of chronic arsenic exposure.[26] Although some people incarcerated in that facility could theoretically purchase uncontaminated bottled water, extremely low pay and regulated income limits for incarcerated people make this alternative water source infeasible.[26]

To evaluate this potential environmental source of health inequity in the context of acutely insufficient national testing data, we investigated possible exposure based on validated approaches to estimating drinking water contamination.[8] We modeled the hydrologically feasible PFAS drinking water exposures for the 6118 carceral facilities in the United States to determine (1) how many incarcerated people are potentially affected, and (2) where testing disparities may lead to underassessments of risk for incarcerated people and, by extension, accountability for PFAS contamination. To achieve these goals we modeled both known contamination sources[27] and, using a newly created and validated method, presumptive contamination sources.[8] We elucidate, to our knowledge, previously unknown drivers of exposure risks faced by a large structurally vulnerable population and indicate priority sites for testing.

METHODS

We conducted geospatial data analysis in R version 4.1.0 (RStudio, Boston, MA) to identify US carceral facilities in the same watershed boundary and, as a proxy for hydrological flow direction, at a lower elevation than point sources with known and likely PFAS contamination.

We identified 6118 US carceral facilities designated as not closed from the Department of Homeland Security (DHS) Prison Boundaries data set.[28] This data set records administrative data, along with polygon geometries of fence lines or building footprints, for secure detention centers in the United States, ranging in jurisdiction from federal facilities (including military facilities) to local governments.

We then identified 1774 known PFAS contamination sites using the PFAS Project Lab's PFAS Contamination Site Tracker.[27] These are locations where environmental monitoring has identified a specific facility or location as having PFAS contamination above laboratory detection or reporting limits. However, known PFAS contamination has been disproportionately identified in states with rigorous testing regimes and thus underrepresents the scope of contamination. Unrepresentative testing is compounded by historically high detection and reporting thresholds, geographically uneven levels of testing, exclusions of private wells from government testing programs, and disincentives to develop and report PFAS testing data in the absence of federal standards and funding.[8]

Therefore, we also identified 57 412 presumptive PFAS contamination sites using the presumptive PFAS contamination model of Salvatore et al.,[8] which identifies locations where contamination is likely and should be assumed in the absence of high-quality testing data to the contrary. This model includes 3 categories of PFAS point sources: sites that release aqueous film–forming foam (including Department of Defense sites, fire training sites, and airports), certain industrial sites, and sites related to PFAS waste (including wastewater treatments plants and landfills). PFASs are a central component of aqueous film–forming foam used in firefighting, which is widely used in suppressing fuel fires and, even more frequently, training exercises. Additionally, PFASs are used in more than 200 categories in industrial or manufacturing processes or finished goods.[29] Wastewater treatment plants and landfills are sources because they concentrate the waste stream PFAS-containing products and PFAS-contaminated water. The validation techniques in Salvatore et al.[8] show high correspondence between known and suspected sites.

We excluded a number of potentially relevant data sources from analysis because of data quality concerns. As of 2020, certain US facilities were required to report certain PFAS emissions via the Toxic Release Inventory. In 2022, 47 facilities reported PFAS emissions to the Toxic Release Inventory. We conducted separate analyses that included these point sources, and changes to our findings were negligible. We excluded this category based on our concern that the recent implementation, combined with a very small number of actual reported sites, resulted in dramatic underestimations of the total emitted PFASs.[30]

We were unable to include in our analysis data from the EPA's third Unregulated Contaminant Monitoring Rule (UCMR 3), which at the time of our analysis provided the only available nationwide data on PFAS concentration levels reported in public drinking water systems. (The next round of UCMR is ongoing through 2025.) Matching UCMR 3 data at the water system level with point data on carceral facility locations is impossible because there is no nationwide database with geolocation boundaries for all public drinking water systems. By individually checking every carceral facility in the DHS Prison Boundaries data set with EPA's Facility Registration Service, we found that only 383 carceral facilities (< 6%) have their own Safe Drinking Water Information Service ID and therefore their own public water system. Additionally, because UCMR 3 includes only public drinking water systems serving more than 10 000 and a small sample of smaller systems, virtually all carceral drinking water systems would have been excluded from UCMR 3 testing entirely.

Using the US Geological Survey's (USGS's) 12-digit hydrologic unit codes

(HUC-12), we determined the watershed boundaries for all point sources. HUC-12 s designate upstream areas of land that contribute to surface water runoff toward a specific point in a stream or other body of water and represent the smallest watershed subdivisions available via USGS's Watershed Boundary Dataset. We determined elevations for point sources via the USGS Elevation Point Query Service. We then calculated the number, percentage, and populations of carceral facilities colocated with a point source.

Throughout this article, we use the term "colocated" to refer to facilities that are in a HUC-12 with and at a lower elevation than a PFAS point source. We also identified each carceral facility's census block, using the US Census Bureau's TIGERweb API (application programming interface), and we determined whether the facility was in a rural or urban location via census block classification. We disaggregated the results by carceral facility type, whether the facility was a juvenile facility, and whether the facility was in an urban census block. To contextualize the results, we repeated all calculations using the DHS Hospitals data set,[31] which allowed us to determine the percentage of the 8013 US hospitals (excluding nursing homes and health centers) colocated with PFAS point sources.

We selected hospitals as a comparison setting because the number of US hospitals is similar to the number of US carceral facilities, although hospitals house a less racially skewed vulnerable population. Notably, exposure risks in hospitals are likely lower than those in carceral facilities, given that most hospital stays are considerably shorter than detention durations. Additionally, some hospitals use point-of-entry and point-of-use filters for infection prevention, which could mitigate PFAS exposure. The prevalence and PFAS efficacy of these filters has not been studied.

Finally, to determine priority locations for increased PFAS monitoring, we performed a series of statistical tests to determine whether there was a significant difference in proportions of certain carceral facilities near known versus presumptive PFAS contamination sites. Specifically, we determined the proportions of carcerally proximate PFAS sites that were industrial sources (vs nonindustrial) from the corpus of known sites and the corpus of presumptive sites. We used a 2-proportion *z*-test to determine whether there was a statistically significant difference in proportions across the 2 data sources.

To assess the spatial independence of facilities, we ran a spatial bootstrap test based on the Moran I statistic and found the spatial autocorrelation of the type of facilities to be very weak ($I = 0.08$). Our analysis thus assumes that point locations are independent and identically distributed. In addition, for both juvenile and nonjuvenile facilities, we tagged each facility we determined to be colocated with a suspected PFAS contamination source but not a known contamination source as "presumed only." Using a permutation test, we tested the null hypothesis that whether a facility is juvenile or adult makes no difference when it comes to the proportion of facilities where colocation with a PFAS source was presumed only. Permutation tests only presume the exchangeability of observations, an assumption that these data meet.

RESULTS

We found that 310 (5%) active US carceral facilities have at least 1 known source of PFAS contamination in the same watershed boundary and at a higher elevation than the facility (Figure 1). At least 150 000 people are incarcerated in these facilities, including at least 2200 juveniles. Calculations of the size of affected populations are significantly underestimated because 31% of all active carceral facilities are missing population data. Missing population data are biased toward juvenile carceral facilities, with 50% of juvenile carceral facilities missing population data compared with 27% of adult carceral facilities. Proximity to known PFAS contamination sites is likely the tip of the iceberg when it comes to risks of PFAS exposure. Nearly half (47%) of all active US carceral facilities have at least 1 presumptive source of PFAS contamination in the same watershed boundary and at a higher elevation than the facility. At least 990 000 people are incarcerated in those facilities, including at least 12 800 juveniles.

These values are similar to the percentages of hospitals colocated with a source of PFAS contamination: 6% of hospitals are colocated with a known source, and 56% are colocated with a presumptive source. Disaggregating the results by urban versus rural location, we determined that 66% of urban carceral facilities and 24% of nonurban carceral facilities are colocated with a presumptive source, whereas 64% of urban hospitals and 23% or nonurban hospitals are colocated with a presumptive source. This suggests the importance of considering urbanity when investigating facilities' PFAS exposure risks.

Many carceral facilities face cumulative PFAS exposures: 1874 (31%) active facilities have more than 1 presumptive source of PFAS contamination in the same watershed boundary and at a higher elevation than the facility, and

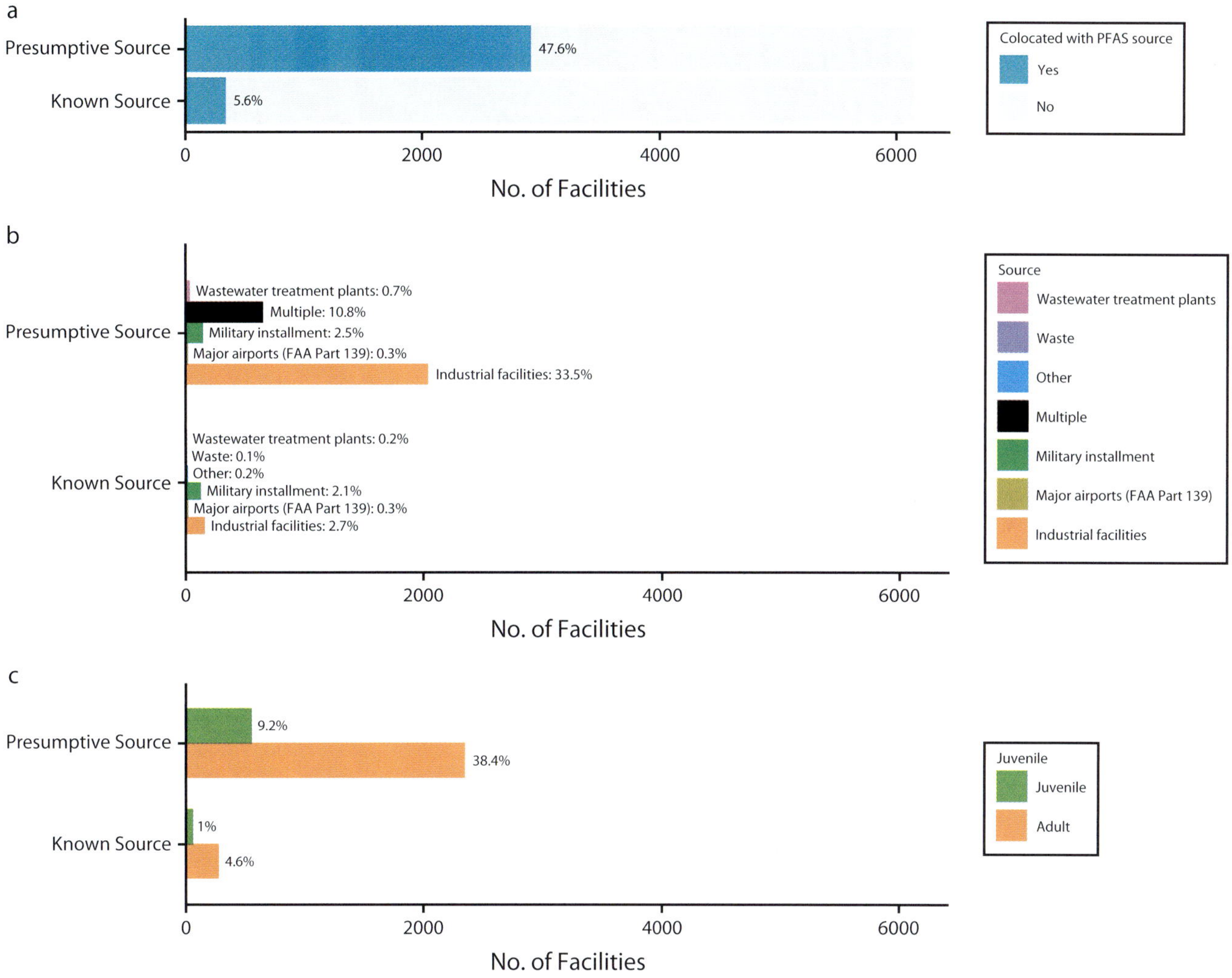

FIGURE 1— Carceral Facilities Colocated With Known and Presumptive Per- and Polyfluoroalkyl Substance (PFAS) Contamination Sources (a) Overall, (b) by Source, and (c) by Juvenile Carceral Facilities: United States, 2022

Note. FAA = Federal Aviation Administration. Percentages indicate the percentage of the total carceral facilities in the same watershed boundary and at a lower elevation than PFAS contamination sites. "Waste" and "other" are not included as categories of presumptive PFAS contamination. "Multiple" is not included as a category of known PFAS contamination.

800 (13%) have more than 5 presumptive sources of PFAS contamination meeting these criteria (Table 1).

Industrial sources are the most frequent presumptive PFAS contamination source to be colocated with carceral facilities (Figure 2), with 2658 (43%) active carceral facilities having at least 1 presumptive PFAS industrial source in the same watershed boundary and at a higher elevation than the facility. Of the presumptive PFAS contamination sources colocated with carceral facilities, 93% were industrial facilities, whereas of the known colocated PFAS contamination sources, 54% were industrial facilities. A *z*-score test indicates a statistically significant difference in proportions across the 2 groups ($P < .01$), highlighting the disproportionate lack of testing at industrial sources compared with other sources, such as military sites and waste sites.

The majority of individuals incarcerated in colocated facilities are in state- and county-run facilities, with at least 480 000 individuals incarcerated in colocated state-run facilities and at least 410 000 in county-run facilities.

Juvenile facilities are disproportionately colocated with presumptive PFAS contamination sites, with 56% of juvenile facilities in the same watershed boundary and at a lower elevation than a presumptive PFAS contamination site and 46% of nonjuvenile facilities meeting these criteria. Furthermore, 65% of locally run juvenile facilities and 62% of county-run juvenile facilities have

TABLE 1— Carceral Facilities in the Same Watershed Boundary and at a Lower Elevation Than Per- and Polyfluoroalkyl Substance (PFAS) Contamination Sites: United States, 2022

Measure	Total Carceral Facilities, No. (%)	Total Carceral Population, No. (Low Estimate)	Juvenile Carceral Facilities, No. (%)	Juvenile Carceral Population (Low Estimate)
Known sources of PFAS contamination				
≤1	310 (5.0)	152 595	57 (5.7)	2 287
2–5	79 (1.3)	32 902	11 (1.1)	460
> 5	10 (0.2)	5 443	3 (0.2)	225
Presumptive sources of PFAS contamination				
≤1	2 885 (47.2)	995 768	558 (55.5)	12 872
2–5	1 874 (30.6)	666 748	394 (39.2)	9 169
> 5	800 (13.1)	327 339	175 (17.4)	4 106

Note. Of all active carceral facilities, 31% were missing population data in the Department of Homeland Security's Prisons Boundaries data set. Percentages in the first column indicate the percentage out of the total carceral facilities in the country. Percentages in the third column indicate the percentage out of the total juvenile carceral facilities in the country.

presumptive PFAS exposure (Figure 3). However, the exposure risks faced by incarcerated youths are also disproportionately underassessed. Via a permutation test, we determined a statistically significant difference ($P<.01$) in the proportion of juvenile versus adult facilities documented as being near a suspected contamination source but not a known contamination source, indicating a need for further testing near juvenile facilities.

DISCUSSION

We found that nearly half of carceral facilities are near at least 1 presumptive PFAS contamination site, suggesting that the incarcerated population potentially faces a major environmental health hazard through their drinking water. By analyzing national data of environmental risks faced by the carceral population, we document the scale of potential exposure risk and inform population health research priorities and interventions. We also found information gaps associated with PFAS contamination to be disproportionate for juvenile carceral facilities and facilities near industrial sources that are presumptive PFAS contamination sources, suggesting the need for targeted testing. These spatial gaps in water monitoring both limit possibilities for regulatory action and mark epistemic inequalities[32] in knowledge investments, as data absences position incarcerated individuals in certain groups and locations to receive less attention from regulators and scientists.

Limitations

Our analysis likely significantly underestimates PFAS exposure potential because the data sets we used to identify known and presumptive contamination are conservative estimates: location of known contamination is biased toward states with rigorous PFAS testing, and the operationalization of presumptive contamination significantly underestimates sites because of limitations in publicly available and geocoded data.[8] In particular, certain states have conducted extensive testing and identified numerous PFAS contamination sites, whereas others have done no focused PFAS testing to date.

Furthermore, our analysis may misestimate drinking water exposure for carceral facilities that receive drinking water sourced from a different watershed, but no nationwide data exist linking carceral facilities' water systems with source locations. It also underestimates potential PFAS exposure by focusing exclusively on drinking water exposures, excluding other known exposure routes, including food, occupation, and inhalation exposures.[33,34] Future research should include exposure investigations of PFAS contamination in carceral facilities, including drinking water and soil sampling, and epidemiological investigations of associated health effects for incarcerated and formerly incarcerated people. Research can also locate existing studies of health status of incarcerated people and determine whether sicker populations are more highly exposed to PFASs.

Public Health Implications

Increased monitoring of carceral facility drinking water is needed to identify the

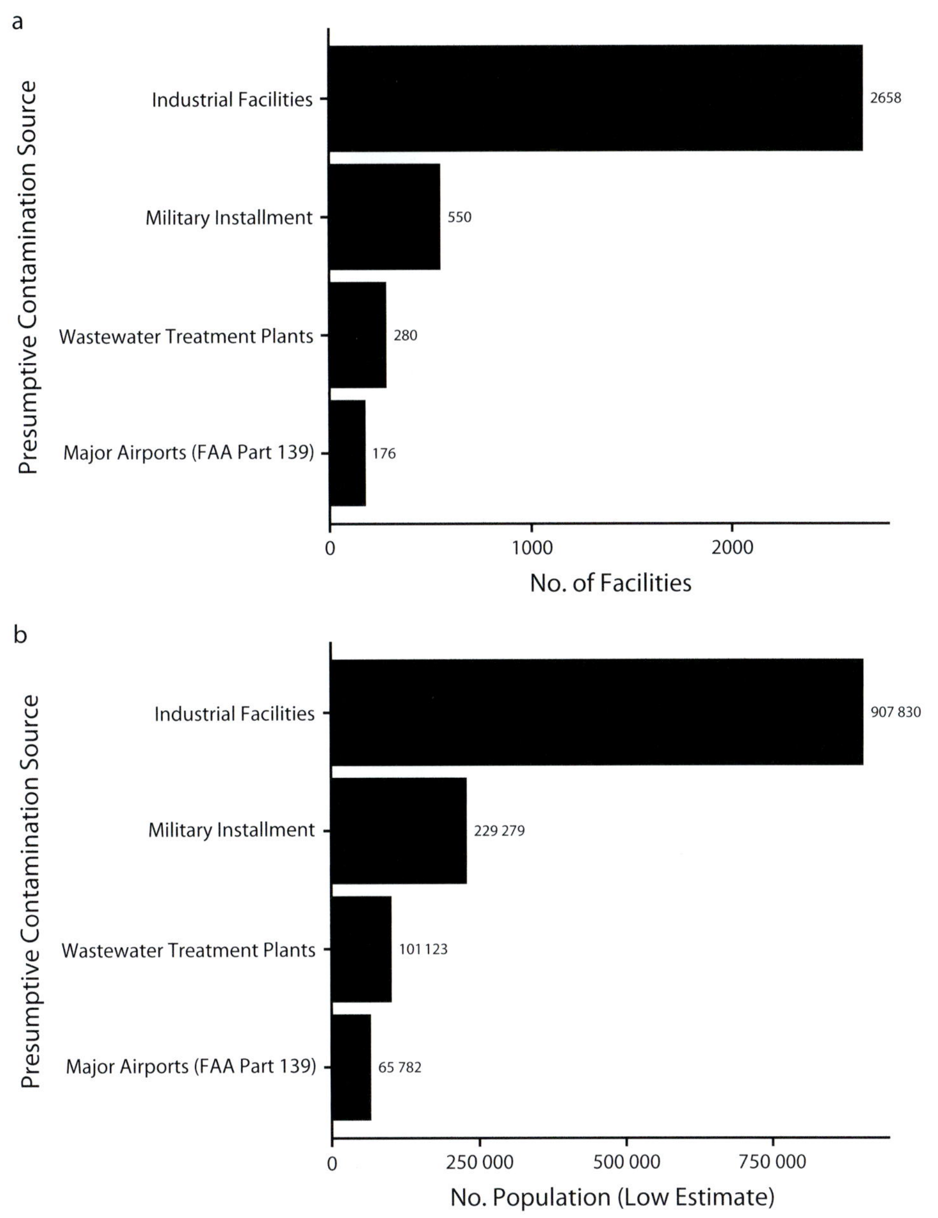

FIGURE 2— Number of (a) Carceral Facilities and (b) Population Colocated with Presumptive Per- and Polyfluoroalkyl Substance (PFAS) Contamination Sources: United States, 2022

Note. FAA = Federal Aviation Administration.

extent of PFAS contamination and potential exposure risk, and testing results should be disclosed to incarcerated populations. If drinking water is contaminated with PFASs above the EPA's proposed maximum contaminant levels, remediation would be required if and when those maximum contaminant levels are finalized. Based on our analysis, in addition to prioritizing testing of water systems serving a large number of individuals, researchers and prison decision-makers should prioritize PFAS testing of drinking water and other media (including soil and food grown onsite) at both juvenile carceral facilities and facilities near known and likely contamination sources.

Partnerships with advocacy groups concerned with carceral health are necessary to ensure that such research is conducted equitably and with meaningful involvement of incarcerated people, their families, and communities hosting

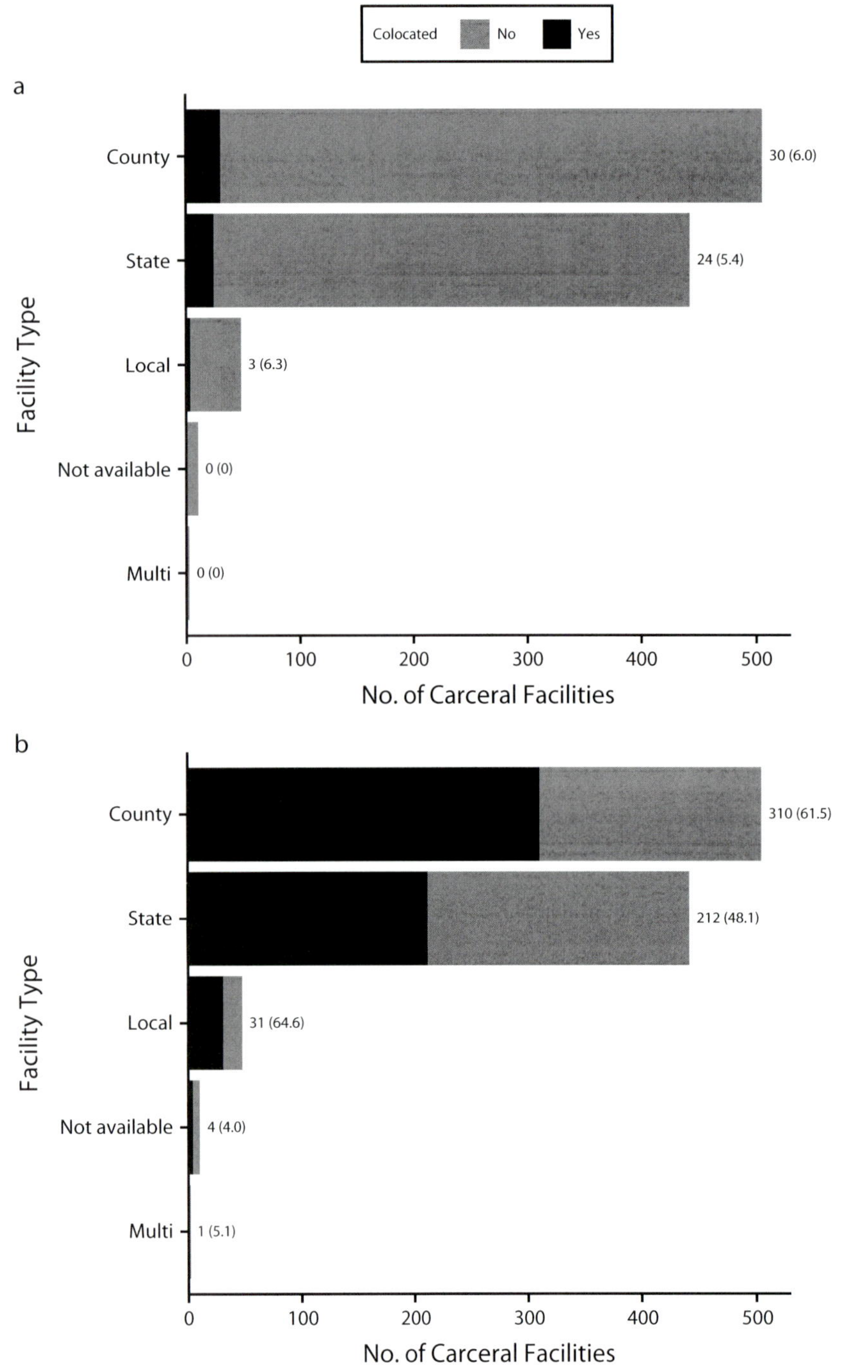

FIGURE 3— **Juvenile Carceral Facilities Colocated With at Least 1 Per- and Polyfluoroalkyl Substance (PFAS) Contamination Source That Is (a) Known, or (b) Presumptive: United States, 2022**

Note. Values to the right of the bars indicate the number of colocated juvenile facilities of the corresponding type with the percentage (in parentheses) of the total juvenile facilities of that type.

carceral facilities. Incarcerated people face structural barriers to raising awareness of the health inequities they face, as well as barriers in obtaining the data, monitoring, and services they need to protect themselves from PFASs and other environmental hazards. This is in stark contrast to the exceptionally rapid and widespread mobilization in the nonincarcerated population of PFAS-affected residents across the United States.

PFASs are immunosuppressants and are associated with increased COVID-19 severity and mortality.[35] In the tight confines of carceral facilities, which increase respiratory infectious disease transmission, it is imperative to reduce any factors that could exacerbate the hazards of airborne pandemics such as COVID-19. Beyond the acute infectious disease crisis that has swept the world over the past nearly 4 years, the chronic health impacts of incarceration are unequally distributed across race, gender, sexual orientation, and gender identity. The long-term effects from these potential exposures are preventable and contribute to health inequities among those who are incarcerated.

Today's widespread public, scientific, and regulatory attention to PFASs could be parlayed into broader environmental monitoring for imprisoned people. That monitoring can contribute to more attention to the overall health of this population, which is historically neglected and faces heightened likelihood for negative health outcomes. AJPH

ABOUT THE AUTHORS

Lindsay Poirier is with the Statistical and Data Sciences Program, Smith College, Northampton, MA. Derrick Salvatore was with the Department of Marine and Environmental Sciences, Northeastern University, Boston, MA. Phil Brown is with the Department of Sociology and Anthropology and Department of Health Sciences, Northeastern University. Alissa Cordner is with the Department of Sociology, Whitman College, Walla Walla, WA. Kira Mok was with the Department of Sociology and Anthropology, Northeastern University. Nicholas Shapiro is with the Institute for Society and Genetics, University of California, Los Angeles.

CORRESPONDENCE

Correspondence should be sent to Lindsay Poirier, Clark Science Center, Smith College, 44 College Ln (100 Green St), Northampton, MA 01063 (e-mail: lpoirier@smith.edu). Reprints can be ordered at http://www.ajph.org by clicking the "Reprints" link.

PUBLICATION INFORMATION

Full Citation: Poirier L, Salvatore D, Brown P, Cordner A, Mok K, Shapiro N. Per- and polyfluoroalkyl substance exposure risks in US carceral facilities, 2022. *Am J Public Health*. 2024;114(5):501–510.

Acceptance Date: December 22, 2023.

DOI: https://doi.org/10.2105/AJPH.2024.307571

CONTRIBUTORS

L. Poirier led data analysis. L. Poirier and N. Shapiro conceptualized the study. D. Salvatore, P. Brown, A. Cordner, and K. Mok were responsible for data curation and validation. All authors collaboratively developed the methodology for this study and contributed to writing, reviewing, and editing.

ACKNOWLEDGMENTS

Aspects of this work were supported by the National Science Foundation (grants SES-1456897 and SES-2120510) and the Robert Wood Johnson Foundation (grant 79111).

In memory of Kenneth Johnson and his insights on carceral drinking water issues. The authors thank the Carceral Ecologies Lab (University of California, Los Angeles), the PFAS Project Lab (Northeastern University and Whitman College), and the Data Ethnography and Advocacy Lab (Smith College) for their collective insights. Thanks are due to Neal Fultz and Kaitlyn Cook for statistical consultations and Alli Morgan and Juniper Huang for support in article preparation.

Note. The content of this article is solely the responsibility of the authors and does not necessarily represent the official views of the funders that provided support for this research.

CONFLICTS OF INTEREST

The authors have no conflicts of interest to disclose.

HUMAN PARTICIPANT PROTECTION

No protocol approval was necessary because this study did not involve human participants.

REFERENCES

1. US Environmental Protection Agency. PFAS strategic roadmap: EPA's commitments to action 2021–2024. June 29, 2022. Available at: https://www.epa.gov/pfas/pfas-strategic-roadmap-epas-commitments-action-2021-2024. Accessed August 11, 2022.
2. Interstate Technology and Regulatory Council. PFAS—per- and polyfluoroalkyl substances fact sheets. Available at: https://pfas-1.itrcweb.org/fact-sheets. Accessed August 7, 2023.
3. National PFAS Contamination Coalition. Available at: https://pfasproject.net. Accessed August 7, 2023.
4. Friedman L, Giang V. 3M reaches $10.3 billion settlement in "forever chemicals" suits. *New York Times*. June 22, 2023. Available at: https://www.nytimes.com/2023/06/22/business/3m-settlement-forever-chemicals-lawsuit.html. Accessed August 11, 2023.
5. Brinkley-Rubinstein L, Cloud DH. Invited perspective: uncovering harmful exposures in carceral environments. *Environ Health Perspect*. 2022;130(9):91305. https://doi.org/10.1289/EHP11653
6. Pellow DN. *What Is Critical Environmental Justice?* Cambridge, UK: Polity; 2017.
7. Wildeman C. Incarceration and population health in wealthy democracies*. *Criminology*. 2016;54(2):360–382. https://doi.org/10.1111/1745-9125.12107
8. Salvatore D, Mok K, Garrett KK, et al. Presumptive contamination: a new approach to PFAS contamination based on likely sources. *Environ Sci Technol Lett*. 2022;9(11):983–990. https://doi.org/10.1021/acs.estlett.2c00502
9. Environmental Protection Agency. Our current understanding of the human health and environmental risks of PFAS. October 14, 2021. Available at: https://www.epa.gov/pfas/our-current-understanding-human-health-and-environmental-risks-pfas. Accessed December 8, 2021.
10. Andrews DQ, Naidenko OV. Population-wide exposure to per- and polyfluoroalkyl substances from drinking water in the United States. *Environ Sci Technol Lett*. 2020;7(12):931–936. https://doi.org/10.1021/acs.estlett.0c00713
11. US Environmental Protection Agency. Per- and polyfluoroalkyl substances (PFAS): proposed PFAS national primary drinking water regulation. 2023. Available at: https://www.epa.gov/sdwa/and-polyfluoroalkyl-substances-pfas. Accessed August 24, 2023.
12. Sawyer W, Wagner P. Mass incarceration: the whole pie 2022. March 14, 2022. Available at: https://www.prisonpolicy.org/reports/pie2022.html. Accessed February 5, 2023.
13. Zeng Z, Minton TD. Jail inmates in 2019. March 2021. Available at: https://bjs.ojp.gov/content/pub/pdf/ji19.pdf. Accessed February 18, 2023.
14. Brinkley-Rubinstein L, Cloud DH. Mass incarceration as a social-structural driver of health inequities: a supplement to *AJPH*. *Am J Public Health*. 2020;110(suppl 1):S14–S15. https://doi.org/10.2105/AJPH.2019.305486
15. Patterson EJ. The dose–response of time served in prison on mortality: New York State, 1989–2003. *Am J Public Health*. 2013;103(3):523–528. https://doi.org/10.2105/AJPH.2012.301148
16. Link NW, Ward JT, Stansfield R. Consequences of mental and physical health for reentry and recidivism: toward a health-based model of desistance*. *Criminology*. 2019;57(3):544–573. https://doi.org/10.1111/1745-9125.12213
17. Barnert ES, Dudovitz R, Nelson BB, et al. How does incarcerating young people affect their adult health outcomes? *Pediatrics*. 2017;139(2):e20162624. https://doi.org/10.1542/peds.2016-2624
18. Center for American Progress. Unjust: LBGT youths incarcerated in the juvenile justice system. June 2017. Available at: https://www.lgbtmap.org/file/lgbtq-incarcerated-youth.pdf. Accessed August 11, 2023.
19. Lambie I, Randell I. The impact of incarceration on juvenile offenders. *Clin Psychol Rev*. 2013;33(3):448–459. https://doi.org/10.1016/j.cpr.2013.01.007
20. American Public Health Association. Advancing public health interventions to address the harms of the carceral system. October 24, 2020. Available at: https://www.apha.org/policies-and-advocacy/public-health-policy-statements/policy-database/2021/01/14/advancing-public-health-interventions-to-address-the-harms-of-the-carceral-system. Accessed February 15, 2023.
21. Toman EL. Something in the air: toxic pollution in and around US prisons. *Punishm Soc*. 2023;25(4):867–887. https://doi.org/10.1177/14624745221114826
22. Skarha J, Spangler K, Dosa D, Rich JD, Savitz DA, Zanobetti A. Heat-related mortality in US state and private prisons: a case-crossover analysis. *PLoS One*. 2023;18(3):e0281389. https://doi.org/10.1371/journal.pone.0281389
23. Connor G. An investigation and analysis of environmental problems at prisons. *Natl Enviromental Enforc J*. 2003;18(4):3–7. Available at: https://nationinside.org/wp-content/uploads/2016/04/EPA_2003_Prison_Initiative_article_original.pdf. Accessed August 11, 2023.
24. Rich JD, Chandler R, Williams BA, et al. How health care reform can transform the health of criminal justice–involved individuals. *Health Aff (Millwood)*. 2014;33(3):462–467. https://doi.org/10.1377/hlthaff.2013.1133
25. Nigra AE, Navas-Acien A. Arsenic in US correctional facility drinking water, 2006–2011. *Environ Res*. 2020;188:109768. https://doi.org/10.1016/j.envres.2020.109768
26. Rempel J, Ray I, Hessl E, et al. The human right to water: a 20-year comparative analysis of arsenic in rural and carceral drinking water systems in California. *Environ Health Perspect*. 2022;130(9):97701. https://doi.org/10.1289/EHP10758
27. PFAS Project Lab. PFAS contamination site tracker. June 2022. Available at: https://pfasproject.com/pfas-sites-and-community-resources. Accessed August 11, 2022.
28. Department of Homeland Security. Homeland Infrastructure Foundation level data (HIFLD). Prison boundaries. July 7, 2020. Available at: https://hifld-geoplatform.opendata.arcgis.com/datasets/geoplatform::prison-boundaries/about. Accessed August 11, 2022.
29. Glüge J, Scheringer M, Cousins IT, et al. An overview of the uses of per- and polyfluoroalkyl substances (PFAS). *Environ Sci Process Impacts*. 2020;22(12):2345–2373. https://doi.org/10.1039/d0em00291g
30. Yiliqi, Reade A. New EPA data: huge amounts of PFAS underreported and burned. October 21, 2021. Available at: https://www.nrdc.org/experts/yiliqi/new-epa-data-huge-amounts-pfas-underreported-and-burned-0. Accessed August 11, 2022.
31. Department of Homeland Security. Homeland Infrastructure Foundation Level Data (HIFLD). Hospitals. June 27, 2023. Available at: https://hifld-geoplatform.opendata.arcgis.com/datasets/7507

9bdea94743bcaca7b6e833692639_0/explore?location=41.335195%2C-147.890230%2C4.62. Accessed June 27, 2023.

32. Kinchy A, Parks S, Jalbert K. Fractured knowledge: mapping the gaps in public and private water monitoring efforts in areas affected by shale gas development. *Environ Plan C Gov Policy.* 2016; 34(5):879–899. https://doi.org/10.1177/0263774X15614684

33. Lucas K, Gaines LGT, Paris-Davila T, Nylander-French LA. Occupational exposure and serum levels of per- and polyfluoroalkyl substances (PFAS): a review. *Am J Ind Med.* 2023;66(5): 379–392. https://doi.org/10.1002/ajim.23454

34. Li J, Sun J, Li P. Exposure routes, bioaccumulation and toxic effects of per- and polyfluoroalkyl substances (PFASs) on plants: a critical review. *Environ Int.* 2022;158:106891. https://doi.org/10.1016/j.envint.2021.106891

35. Grandjean P, Timmermann CAG, Kruse M, et al. Severity of COVID-19 at elevated exposure to perfluorinated alkylates. *PLoS One.* 2020;15(12): e0244815. https://doi.org/10.1371/journal.pone.0244815

Trajectories of Mental Distress Among US Women by Sexual Orientation and Racialized Group During the First Year of the COVID-19 Pandemic

Ariel L. Beccia, PhD, Dougie Zubizarreta, SM, S. Bryn Austin, ScD, SM, Julia R. Raifman, ScD, SM, Jorge E. Chavarro, MD, ScD, SM, and Brittany M. Charlton, ScD, SM

Objectives. To describe longitudinal trends in the prevalence of mental distress across the first year of the COVID-19 pandemic (April 2020–April 2021) among US women at the intersection of sexual orientation and racialized group.

Methods. Participants included 49 805 cisgender women and female-identified people from the COVID-19 Sub-Study, a cohort of US adults embedded within the Nurses' Health Studies 2 and 3 and the Growing Up Today Study. We fit generalized estimating equation Poisson models to estimate trends in depressive and anxiety symptoms by sexual orientation (gay or lesbian, bisexual, mostly heterosexual, completely heterosexual); subsequent models explored further differences by racialized group (Asian, Black, Latine, White, other or unlisted).

Results. Relative to completely heterosexual peers, gay or lesbian, bisexual, and mostly heterosexual women had a higher prevalence of depressive and anxiety symptoms at each study wave and experienced widening inequities over time. Inequities were largest for sexual minority women of color, although confidence intervals were wide.

Conclusions. The COVID-19 pandemic may have exacerbated already-glaring mental health inequities affecting sexual minority women, especially those belonging to marginalized racialized groups. Future research should investigate structural drivers of these patterns to inform policy-oriented interventions.
(*Am J Public Health*. 2024;114(5):511–522. https://doi.org/10.2105/AJPH.2024.307601)

AJPH May 2024, Vol. 114, No. 5

The COVID-19 pandemic has had a profound negative impact on mental health in the United States, including by exacerbating long-standing inequities experienced by structurally marginalized populations. Sexual orientation–related inequities (i.e., those rooted in heterosexism and affecting lesbian, gay, bisexual, and other sexual minority groups) have been particularly amplified.[1] For example, nationally representative data reveal how sexual minorities were more than twice as likely as heterosexuals to report depression and anxiety in March and April of 2020[2,3]; there is also evidence that the increases in mental distress observed pre- to post-pandemic onset of the COVID-19 pandemic within the general US population were significantly larger among sexual minority groups.[4,5] These patterns hold concerning implications for health justice, and they underscore the urgent need to consider sexual minority mental health within COVID-19 relief efforts and in response to future crises.

However, attributable in part to the systematic erasure of sexual minorities within public health surveillance systems,[6] critical knowledge gaps remain that are hindering action. First, it is largely unknown whether the inequities observed at the start of the pandemic have attenuated, persisted, or even widened over time—information needed to guide resource allocation and intervention development. We are aware of only 2 studies that used prospectively collected longitudinal data to examine changes in mental distress prevalence by sexual orientation from early to late 2020[7,8]; other studies aiming to assess such trends have relied on data collected at a single point in time,[9] which can be subject to recall bias and cannot capture long-term fluctuations.

Second, despite substantial evidence regarding the gendered nature of the pandemic (e.g., increased domestic loads, financial strain, and exposure to violence for individuals from marginalized gender groups),[10] very few studies have focused on elucidating the potentially unique mental health experiences of sexual minority women. Extant research has mostly analyzed sexual minority participants of all genders together within umbrella lesbian, gay, bisexual, transgender, and queer (LGBTQ+) categories,[11,12] likely because of small samples; yet, available studies that have been able to disaggregate by both sexual orientation and gender point to subgroup differences, including pronounced inequities for lesbian and bisexual women.[5,13] Additional research is needed to further parse out these patterns.

Finally, there continues to be a concerning lack of data on pandemic-related mental health at the intersection of sexual orientation, gender, and other dimensions of social position, most notably race and ethnicity. The disproportionate negative impacts of the pandemic on marginalized racialized groups in the United States as a result of historical and ongoing forms of structural racism (e.g., residential segregation) are widely documented,[14,15] and numerous studies reveal how such impacts have contributed to elevated depression and anxiety and exacerbated mental health inequities for Asian, Black, and Latine people.[16,17] Moreover, research from Europe has found that sexual minority women of color experienced especially high levels of mental distress during early pandemic waves,[18] which is suggestive of compounded patterns of risk for multiply marginalized communities. However, whether the same is true in the United States and, more generally, how the pandemic has impacted mental health across diverse population subgroups over time, is understudied.

We sought to address these gaps by examining changes in mental distress over the first year of the pandemic among US women across intersections of sexual orientation and racialized group. Using data from a cohort of cisgender women and female-identified people, we aimed to (1) describe longitudinal trends in the prevalence of depressive and anxiety symptoms from April 2020 to April 2021, (2) identify and quantify the magnitude of sexual orientation–related inequities, and (3) explore further heterogeneity by racialized group. Our analyses were informed by the minority stress model,[19–21] a leading theory of sexual minority health that situates sexual orientation–related inequities in relation to heterosexist stigma and discrimination and recognizes the likelihood of differential stigma and discrimination experiences and resultant mental health outcomes across sexual minority subgroups (e.g., lesbian vs bisexual women); accordingly, we formulated our models to obtain subgroup-specific estimates and interpreted our findings as reflecting the downstream impact of relevant social stressors. For our exploratory third aim, we additionally drew on the Black feminist principle of intersectionality,[22–24] which highlights the interconnected nature of heterosexism with other systems of power (e.g., sexism, racism), in turn emphasizing the need to examine population health patterns along multiple axes of social position simultaneously.[25] Taken together, our theoretically guided analyses allow us to build on the extant literature and provide new knowledge on how the pandemic has shaped population mental health and mental health inequities in the United States.

METHODS

We used data from the COVID-19 Sub-Study,[26] a US-based cohort embedded within the Nurses' Health Studies 2 (NHS2) and 3 (NHS3) and the Growing Up Today Study (GUTS). Baseline surveys were completed by 58 612 of 105 662 invited participants in April 2020; follow-ups were administered monthly and then quarterly (7 total study waves). Because NHS2, NHS3, and GUTS originally enrolled registered or in-training nurses and their families,[27] a sizeable proportion of participants in the COVID-19 Sub-Study are current or previous health care workers and are predominantly White and middle- to upper-middle-class. Further details about these cohorts are provided elsewhere.[26,27]

For the current study, we restricted inclusion to 56 483 cisgender women and female-identified participants (hereafter sometimes referred to as "women"; see Appendix A, available as a supplement to the online version of this article at https://ajph.org, for details on gender measurement). We excluded those who lived outside the United States (n = 747), as such individuals likely had unique experiences with pandemic stressors and resultant mental health outcomes. We subsequently excluded those with missing data on sexual orientation (n = 4395), racialized group (n = 142), or covariates (n = 1375), as well as those who never responded to the relevant outcome measures (n = 246). Our final analytic sample size was 49 805.

Measures

Sexual orientation was assessed at multiple waves of NHS2, NHS3, and GUTS data collection using an item capturing sexual identity and attraction, with response options including "completely heterosexual (attracted to persons of the opposite sex)," "mostly heterosexual," "bisexual (equally attracted to men and women)," "mostly homosexual," "completely homosexual (attracted to persons of the same sex)," or "unsure."[28] To limit misclassification from sexual fluidity, we took participants' report of their sexual orientation from the survey administered closest in time to the start of the pandemic (2017 for NHS2, 2019 for NHS3 and GUTS) and defined 4 categories: completely heterosexual, mostly heterosexual, bisexual, and gay or lesbian (derived by combining mostly and completely homosexual). Unsure respondents were excluded because of small sample sizes.

Our outcomes included depressive and anxiety symptoms, which were assessed at all 7 study waves using the Patient Health Questionnaire (PHQ-2) and the Generalized Anxiety Disorder Scale (GAD-2), respectively.[29,30] These measures follow a similar structure, in that they ask participants to indicate how often they experienced a given symptom during the past week on a 4-point scale. A total score is generated by summing responses to the included items (range = 0–6); we used a cutpoint of 3 to identify participants exhibiting clinically meaningful depressive or anxiety symptoms.[29,30]

We identified a set of adjustment variables inclusive of factors that differed by sexual orientation and were associated with our outcomes but were not hypothesized mediators: cohort (NHS2, NHS3, GUTS), age in years, and US Census region of residence (Northeast, Midwest, South, West, US territory). Racialized group (Asian, Black, Latine, White, other or unlisted) was treated as an effect measure modifier in our exploratory analyses. To further describe the sample, we additionally provide information on participants' occupation, household income, and experiences with pandemic-related financial strain.

Analysis

We started by describing the analytic sample with respect to all variables, overall and by sexual orientation. We then assessed whether the prevalence of depressive and anxiety symptoms differed by sexual orientation or racialized group at each study wave with the χ^2 test.

For our primary analyses, we fit generalized estimating equation Poisson models with an exchangeable correlation matrix to examine longitudinal trends in the prevalence of our mental distress outcomes.[31] Model 1 used study wave as the predictor and estimated its association with a given outcome to obtain prevalence trajectories for the full sample; model 2 used sexual orientation as the predictor and omitted study wave to identify and quantify time-averaged inequities between gay or lesbian, bisexual, or mostly heterosexual participants and the completely heterosexual referent; and model 3 introduced sexual-orientation-by-study-wave interactions to test whether the magnitude of inequities changed over the study period. All models adjusted for cohort, age, and Census region and were weighted by the inverse of the probability of being censored at a given study wave (see Appendix B, available as a supplement to the online version of this article at https://ajph.org). We summarized results by using prevalence ratios (PRs) and 95% confidence intervals (CIs), as well as predicted probabilities.

We also conducted an exploratory analysis to examine whether prevalence trajectories varied simultaneously along axes of sexual orientation and racialized group. As previously explained, the COVID-19 Sub-Study is predominantly White and middle- to upper-middle-class (as well as cisgender and heterosexual), which limited our ability to comprehensively investigate intersectional inequities. That being said, more than 3000 participants belonged to a marginalized racialized group—including 400 who were also sexual minorities—and intersectional data on pandemic-related mental distress remain sparce. As such, we believed it was important to reveal the experiences of these multiply marginalized subgroups to the extent possible given our sample size constraints. We started by constructing 2 versions of a joint sexual orientation–racialized group variable, one with 8 categories defined by all combinations of sexual orientation and a binarized version of racialized group (marginalized racialized groups [Asian, Black, Latine, and other or unlisted] vs White) and one with 10 categories defined by all combinations of racialized group and a binarized version of sexual orientation (sexual minorities [gay or lesbian, bisexual, and mostly heterosexual] vs completely heterosexual). We then fit a second series of generalized estimating equation Poisson models (using the same covariates and inverse probability weights as described previously): model 4 mirrored model 2 by including the 8-category joint variable as the primary predictor to identify and quantify time-averaged inequities across the relevant intersectional positions; model 5 mirrored model 3 by introducing joint-variable-by-study-wave interactions; and models 6 and 7 mirrored models 4 and 5, respectively, by replacing the 8-category joint variable with the 10-category one.

RESULTS

Characteristics of the analytic sample are presented in Table 1. Most participants were White women from NHS2 who were either working full-time or retired and had a household income of \$50 001 to \$100 000. Their mean age was 57.6 years, with sexual minority participants (i.e., those identifying as mostly heterosexual, bisexual, or gay or lesbian) being slightly younger than those identifying as completely heterosexual. Although levels of unemployment and pandemic-related financial strain were relatively low in the full sample, these experiences were more common for sexual minorities. Furthermore, mostly heterosexual, bisexual, and gay or lesbian participants were all significantly more likely than completely heterosexual peers to report depressive and anxiety symptoms at each study wave (Table A, available as a supplement to the online version of this article at https://ajph.org). The distribution of these outcomes by racialized group was less clearly patterned, with some marginalized racialized groups (Latine, other or unlisted) having higher prevalences than White participants and other such groups (Asian, Black) having lower prevalences (Table B, available as a supplement to the online version of this article at https://ajph.org).

Results from our primary analyses are presented in Table 2 and Table C (available as a supplement to the online version of this article at https://ajph.org). In models estimating mental distress trajectories for the full sample, PRs for study wave indicated that the prevalence of depressive symptoms was highest in April 2020 and then subsequently decreased, whereas the prevalence of anxiety symptoms fluctuated across the study period and peaked in October 2020 (Table C, Model 1; Figure 1a). There were considerable inequities by sexual orientation when considering average differences from April 2020 to April 2021, with sexual minorities having a 51% to 95% higher prevalence of depressive symptoms and a 40% to 56% higher prevalence of anxiety symptoms compared with completely heterosexuals; inequities in both outcomes were largest for bisexual participants (Table C, Model 2). Most sexual-orientation-by-study-wave interactions were nonsignificant, indicating that the magnitude of inequities remained stable over time, apart from periodic widenings in depressive symptom inequities for mostly heterosexual and bisexual participants and in anxiety symptom inequities for mostly heterosexual and gay or lesbian participants (Table 2; Figure 1b).

Our exploratory analyses provide evidence of further heterogeneity by racialized group. Given the noted differences in mental distress between Asian, Black, Latine, and other or unlisted racialized groups in relation to White participants, we focus here on results from models using the 10-category joint variable that kept racialized groups disaggregated. Considering first the models examining time-averaged differences (Table D, Model 6, available as a supplement to the online version of this article at https://ajph.org), we found that White sexual minorities, Latine sexual minorities, and sexual minorities belonging to an other or unlisted racialized group had significantly higher prevalences of depressive and anxiety symptoms compared with White completely heterosexual participants from April 2020 to April 2021; Asian and Black sexual minorities, Latine completely heterosexual participants, and completely heterosexual participants belonging to an other or unlisted racialized group had PRs suggestive of similar inequities, although CIs were wide. As indicated by the interaction models (Table D, Model 7; Figure 2), the magnitude of inequities fluctuated across the study period, with several intersectional positions inclusive of multiply marginalized participants (e.g., Black and Latine sexual minorities) experiencing widening inequities over time. Results from models using the 8-category joint variable are given in Table E (available as a supplement to the online version of this article at https://ajph.org).

DISCUSSION

Our results reveal concerning mental health inequities among US sexual minority women that either persisted or widened in magnitude during the first year of the COVID-19 pandemic. Consistent with previous work,[2–5] we found that gay or lesbian, bisexual, and mostly heterosexual participants reported higher levels of depressive and anxiety

TABLE 1— Baseline Sociodemographic Characteristics of the Cisgender Women and Female-Identified Participants in the COVID-19 Sub-Study: United States, April 2020

	Full Sample (n = 49 805), No. (%) or Mean ±SD	Completely Heterosexual (n = 45 299), No. (%) or Mean ±SD	Mostly Heterosexual (n = 3262), No. (%) or Mean ±SD	Bisexual (n = 559), No. (%) or Mean ±SD	Gay or Lesbian (n = 685), No. (%) or Mean ±SD
Cohort					
Nurses' Health Study 2	35 352 (71.0)	33 768 (74.5)	1 022 (31.3)	172 (30.8)	390 (56.9)
Nurses' Health Study 3	10 097 (20.3)	8 356 (18.4)	1 308 (40.1)	228 (40.8)	205 (29.9)
Growing Up Today Study	4 356 (8.7)	3 175 (7.0)	932 (28.6)	159 (28.4)	90 (13.1)
Age, y (range = 21–74 y)[a]	57.6 ± 13.2	58.6 ± 12.6	45.6 ± 14.3	45.6 ± 14.9	54.5 ± 14.3
Racialized group					
Asian	593 (1.2)	546 (1.2)	37 (1.1)	< 10	< 10
Black	496 (1.0)	455 (1.0)	28 (0.9)	< 10	< 10
Latine	1 019 (2.0)	886 (2.0)	91 (2.8)	23 (4.1)	19 (2.8)
White	46 601 (93.6)	42 495 (93.8)	2 985 (91.5)	493 (88.2)	628 (91.7)
Other or unlisted	1 096 (2.2)	917 (2.0)	121 (3.7)	35 (6.3)	23 (3.4)
Census region of residence					
Midwest	14 833 (29.8)	13 792 (30.4)	774 (23.7)	120 (21.5)	147 (21.5)
Northeast	13 505 (27.1)	12 277 (27.1)	887 (27.2)	156 (27.9)	185 (27.0)
South	11 711 (23.5)	10 773 (23.8)	669 (20.5)	106 (19.0)	163 (23.8)
West	9 743 (19.6)	8 445 (18.6)	932 (28.6)	177 (31.7)	189 (27.6)
US territories	13 (0.0)	12 (0.0)	< 10	< 10	< 10
Occupational status[b]					
Working full-time	19 162 (38.5)	16 657 (36.8)	1 842 (56.5)	326 (58.3)	337 (49.2)
Working part-time	7 133 (14.3)	6 441 (14.2)	533 (16.3)	80 (14.3)	79 (11.5)
Volunteering	1 541 (3.1)	1 427 (3.2)	77 (2.4)	14 (2.5)	23 (3.4)
Student	830 (1.7)	606 (1.3)	152 (4.7)	51 (9.1)	21 (3.1)
Military	51 (0.1)	40 (0.1)	< 10	< 10	< 10
Parental leave	246 (0.5)	193 (0.4)	43 (1.3)	< 10	< 10
Staying home with children	2 605 (5.2)	2 244 (5.0)	296 (9.1)	42 (7.5)	23 (3.4)
Retired	19 365 (38.9)	18 568 (41.0)	505 (15.5)	84 (15.0)	208 (30.4)
Retired but working because of pandemic	163 (0.3)	156 (0.3)	< 10	< 10	< 10
Unemployed, laid off, or furloughed	1 643 (3.3)	1 412 (3.1)	168 (5.2)	41 (7.3)	22 (3.2)
Not working because of disability	899 (1.8)	799 (1.8)	55 (1.7)	16 (2.9)	29 (4.2)
Other	1 171 (2.4)	1 072 (2.4)	71 (2.2)	14 (2.5)	14 (2.0)
Current health care worker[c]	19 484 (39.1)	17 382 (38.4)	1 565 (48.0)	257 (46.0)	280 (40.9)
Household income, $[d]					
< 15 000	181 (0.5)	145 (0.5)	20 (1.1)	10 (3.1)	< 10
15 000–30 000	777 (2.3)	605 (2.0)	100 (5.5)	41 (12.7)	31 (7.1)
30 001–50 000	3 705 (11.1)	3 373 (11.0)	212 (11.7)	54 (16.7)	66 (15.1)
50 001–100 000	15 095 (45.3)	14 099 (45.8)	703 (38.9)	116 (35.8)	177 (40.4)
100 001–200 000	8 906 (26.7)	8 130 (26.4)	573 (31.7)	77 (23.8)	126 (28.8)
> 200 000	4 683 (14.0)	4 428 (14.4)	197 (10.9)	26 (8.0)	32 (7.3)
Missing	16 458	14 519	1457	235	247

Continued

TABLE 1— Continued

	Full Sample (n = 49 805), No. (%) or Mean ±SD	Completely Heterosexual (n = 45 299), No. (%) or Mean ±SD	Mostly Heterosexual (n = 3262), No. (%) or Mean ±SD	Bisexual (n = 559), No. (%) or Mean ±SD	Gay or Lesbian (n = 685), No. (%) or Mean ±SD
Pandemic-related financial strain[e]					
Moderate to extreme	2 526 (5.7)	2 142 (5.3)	269 (9.9)	61 (12.9)	54 (9.0)
Missing	5778	5063	540	87	88

Note. All percentages are column percentages and may not sum to 100% because of rounding and non–mutually exclusive categories.
[a]Nurses' Health Study 2 participants were born in years 1947–1964; Nurses' Health Study 3 participants were born in years 1965–2001; and Growing Up Today Study participants were born in years 1982–1995.
[b]Categories are non–mutually exclusive.
[c]Includes currently employed participants who reported working or volunteering within a health care setting and having direct patient contact since March 1, 2020.
[d]Most recently reported in 2001 for the Nurses' Health Study 2, 2010 for the Nurses' Health Study 3, and 2019 for the Growing Up Today Study.
[e]Assessed via an item that asked, "Since the pandemic started, how much of a concern is having enough money for essentials like food and clothing or for paying rent or mortgage?" Those who reported "moderate" to "extreme" concerns were coded as experiencing pandemic-related financial strain.

symptoms compared with completely heterosexual peers from April 2020 to April 2021, with bisexual participants experiencing the widest inequities during this time. Furthermore, our exploratory analyses provide insights into how the pandemic has shaped mental health along intersecting axes of sexual orientation and racialized group, including evidence of pronounced inequities for sexual minority women of color. These findings add nuance to the available longitudinal research on COVID-19–related mental health in the general US population—especially studies finding that early pandemic spikes in mental distress have since attenuated[32]—by revealing how the prevalence of depressive and anxiety symptoms remained high for sexual minority women.

Our guiding theoretical frameworks offer useful interpretations of these patterns. As previously introduced, the minority stress model implicates heterosexist stigma and discrimination in the (re)production of sexual orientation–related mental health inequities,[19–21] with recent work highlighting how the pandemic served to increase sexual minority people's exposure to relevant stressors (e.g., homophobic or biphobic victimization, identity concealment) and amplify their effects. For example, and as revealed by qualitative research,[33,34] sexual minority women faced myriad unique challenges throughout 2020 and 2021 related to their social positioning, including forced time with unsupportive family or housemates during shelter-in-place orders, isolation from the LGBTQ+ community, and rising antiqueer and antifeminist sentiments across mass and social media (as well as within the US government) stemming from the pandemic's divisive politicization. All these experiences could help explain the persistently elevated levels of depressive and anxiety symptoms we observed among mostly heterosexual, bisexual, and gay or lesbian participants, including the spike in anxiety symptoms that occurred in October 2020 during the second major pandemic wave and just before the 2020 presidential election.

Intersectionality extends this perspective by shifting the lens further upstream to consider how structural forms of heterosexism, sexism, and racism may have jointly impacted COVID-19–related mental health outcomes for sexual minority women, and sexual minority women of color specifically. In their essay on intersectional COVID-19 inequities, Pirtle and Wright explain how structural gendered racism (i.e., "the totality of interconnectedness between structural racism and structural sexism") manifested as excess resource insecurity during the pandemic to drive poor outcomes for women of color in the United States.[35(p171)] Such harms were likely further exacerbated for sexual minority women of color because of compounding effects of structural heterosexism, including with respect to this population's increased likelihood of holding essential worker positions and of experiencing job loss or other economic shocks, heteronormativity embedded within COVID-19 containment measures and recovery efforts (e.g., their focus on nuclear or biological families), and a spate of discriminatory anti-LGBTQ+ policies (e.g., "Don't Say Gay" laws) that were introduced and implemented across the United States during the pandemic period.[2,33,34,36,37] Collectively, these

TABLE 2— Longitudinal Trends in the Prevalence of Depressive and Anxiety Symptoms Overall and by Sexual Orientation Among Cisgender Women and Female-Identified Participants in the COVID-19 Sub-Study: United States, April 2020–April 2021

	Depressive Symptoms, PR (95% CI)	Anxiety Symptoms, PR (95% CI)
Study wave		
Baseline/wave 1, Apr 2020	1 (Ref)	1 (Ref)
Wave 2, May 2020	0.84 (0.81, 0.87)	0.90 (0.88, 0.92)
Wave 3, Jun 2020	0.89 (0.86, 0.91)	0.97 (0.95, 1.00)
Wave 4, Jul 2020	0.93 (0.90, 0.96)	1.00 (0.98, 1.03)
Wave 5, Oct 2020	0.97 (0.94, 1.00)	1.14 (1.11, 1.16)
Wave 6, Jan 2021	0.95 (0.92, 0.98)	0.89 (0.87, 0.92)
Wave 7, Apr 2021	0.80 (0.77, 0.82)	0.71 (0.70, 0.73)
Sexual orientation		
Completely heterosexual	1 (Ref)	1 (Ref)
Mostly heterosexual	1.60 (1.49, 1.71)	1.34 (1.27, 1.41)
Bisexual	1.86 (1.63, 2.13)	1.50 (1.36, 1.66)
Gay or lesbian	1.49 (1.27, 1.73)	1.23 (1.09, 1.39)
Study wave x sexual orientation[a]		
Wave 2 × mostly heterosexual	1.08 (0.99, 1.17)	1.10 (1.04, 1.16)
Wave 3 × mostly heterosexual	1.01 (0.93, 1.10)	1.03 (0.97, 1.09)
Wave 4 × mostly heterosexual	1.01 (0.92, 1.10)	1.06 (1.00, 1.12)
Wave 5 × mostly heterosexual	1.10 (1.01, 1.20)	1.07 (1.00, 1.13)
Wave 6 × mostly heterosexual	0.94 (0.86, 1.03)	1.02 (0.95, 1.09)
Wave 7 × mostly heterosexual	1.12 (1.03, 1.22)	1.10 (1.03, 1.18)
Wave 2 × bisexual	1.20 (1.03, 1.40)	1.09 (0.97, 1.24)
Wave 3 × bisexual	1.00 (0.83, 1.19)	1.07 (0.95, 1.21)
Wave 4 × bisexual	0.98 (0.82, 1.16)	1.02 (0.90, 1.16)
Wave 5 × bisexual	1.13 (0.97, 1.32)	1.07 (0.95, 1.20)
Wave 6 × bisexual	0.99 (0.83, 1.17)	1.03 (0.90, 1.19)
Wave 7 × bisexual	1.05 (0.88, 1.25)	0.94 (0.80, 1.11)
Wave 2 × gay or lesbian	1.11 (0.92, 1.34)	1.12 (0.98, 1.29)
Wave 3 × gay or lesbian	0.92 (0.74, 1.14)	1.08 (0.94, 1.24)
Wave 4 × gay or lesbian	1.00 (0.83, 1.21)	1.07 (0.93, 1.24)
Wave 5 × gay or lesbian	1.11 (0.93, 1.32)	1.21 (1.06, 1.39)
Wave 6 × gay or lesbian	1.09 (0.91, 1.30)	1.25 (1.08, 1.45)
Wave 7 × gay or lesbian	0.85 (0.69, 1.06)	1.26 (1.08, 1.48)

Note. CI = confidence interval; PR = prevalence ratio. Results from generalized estimating equation Poisson models. All models are adjusted for cohort, age, and Census region and were weighted to account for loss to follow up and item nonresponse.
[a]Interaction estimates are ratios of prevalence ratios (e.g., the prevalence ratio for mostly heterosexuals vs completely heterosexuals at wave 2/the prevalence ratio for mostly heterosexuals vs completely heterosexuals at wave 1).

ongoing macro-level stressors that uniquely or disproportionately affected multiply marginalized populations could underlie our findings of heightened COVID-19–related mental distress throughout 2020 and 2021 for sexual minority women of color. That being said, we urge caution in drawing conclusions from our exploratory analyses given the following limitations and emphasize the need for further work examining these patterns.

Limitations

As discussed, the COVID-19 Sub-Study is not representative, and its participants are predominantly White women of middle- to upper-middle-class standing.

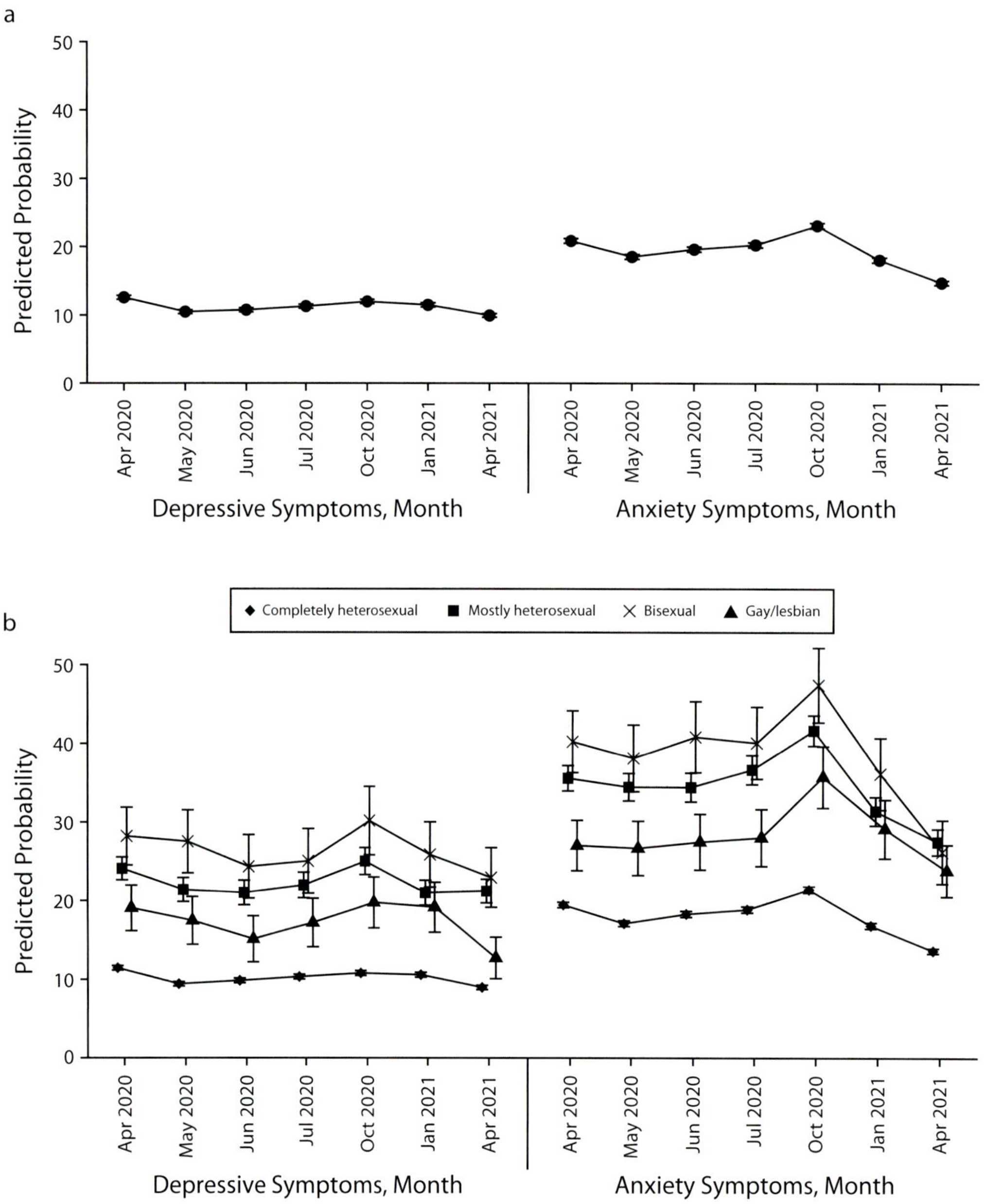

FIGURE 1— **Trajectories of Depressive and Anxiety Symptoms Among Cisgender Women and Female-Identified Participants in the COVID-19 Sub-Study (a) Overall and (b) by Sexual Orientation: United States, April 2020–April 2021**

Moreover, the relatively small sample sizes across Asian, Black, Latine, and other or unlisted racialized groups, coupled with the suboptimal measurement of additional axes of social position (especially gender), precluded our ability to conduct more nuanced intersectional analyses. As such, and in light of the disproportionate impact that the pandemic has had on marginalized racialized groups, transgender or nonbinary people, and low-income and working-class communities, our findings may not generalize.

Second, we were unable to fully explore spatial heterogeneity in our outcomes given data sparsity within small geographic areas (e.g., counties). Studies have documented important differences in pandemic-related mental distress across US geographies as a result of varying public health policies, provision of social safety nets, and access to services[38–40]; our approach of controlling for Census region will likely have obscured these patterns (including how they intersected with those by sexual orientation and racialized group)

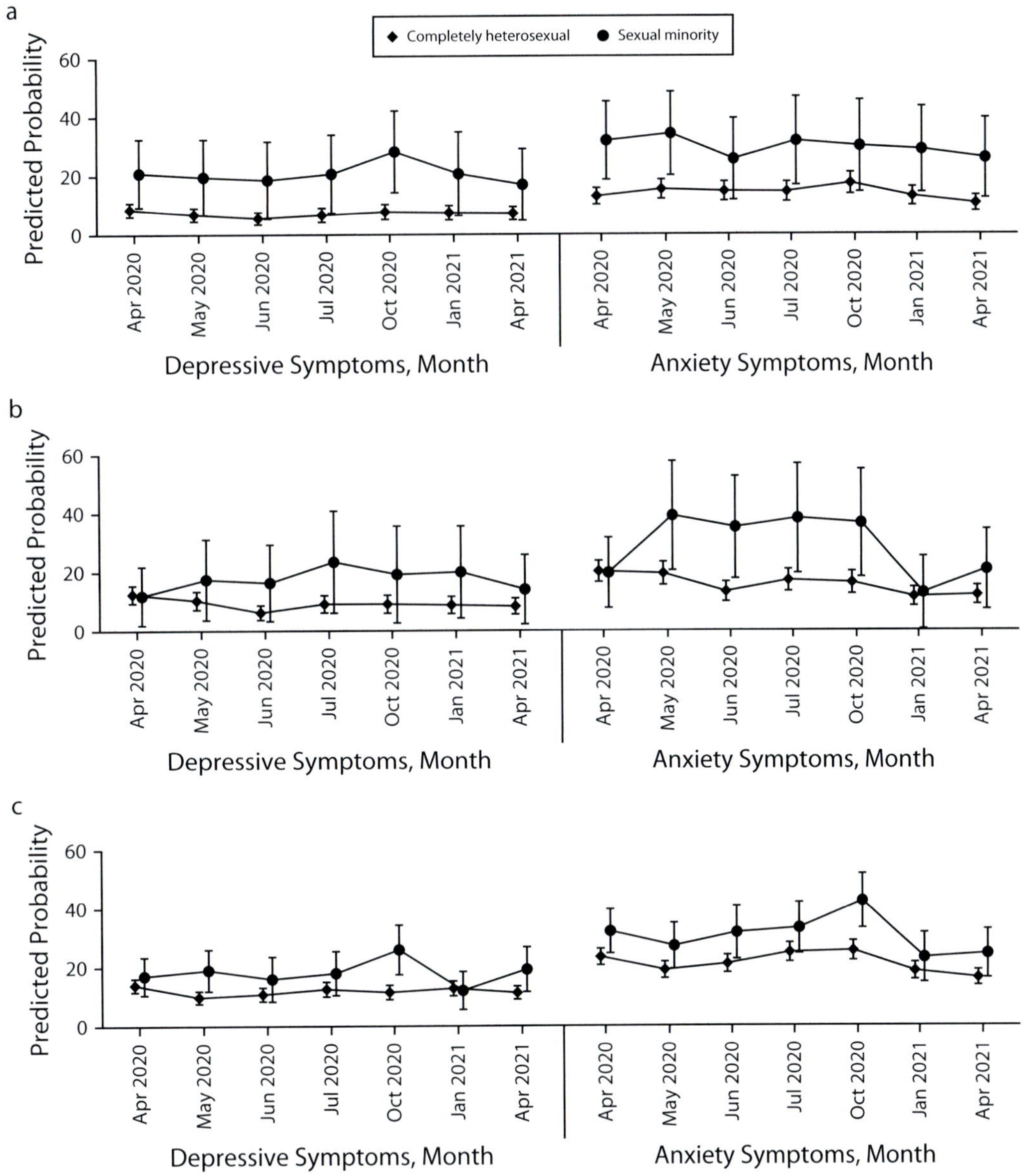

FIGURE 2— **Trajectories of Depressive and Anxiety Symptoms Among Cisgender Women and Female-Identified Participants in the COVID-19 Sub-Study by Intersecting Sexual Orientation and (a) Asian Participants, (b) Black Participants, and (c) Hispanic/Latine Participants: United States, April 2020–April 2021**

Note. For a full figure showing all racialized groups, see Figure A (available as a supplement to the online version of this article at https://ajph.org).

and may have resulted in residual confounding.

Third, although our study period captured a key timeframe that included 3 pandemic surges and numerous sociopolitical events relevant to the health and well-being of US sexual minority women, especially sexual minority women of color (e.g., an upsurge of Black Lives Matter protests in response to ongoing police violence, the 2020 presidential election, and the onslaught of anti-LGBTQ+ legislation), there have been further shifts throughout 2022 to 2023 that likely continued to impact population mental health in complex ways. It will be important for future studies to address these limitations by recruiting diverse, representative, and geographically granular samples and to investigate the multilevel determinants of the inequities we observed.

Public Health Implications

Our study offers several implications for public health practice. First, there is a critical need for enhanced collection of data on sexual orientation and gender identity (SOGI) within local, state, and federal public health surveillance systems.[41,42] Despite early evidence of disproportionate pandemic impacts on LGBTQ+ communities,[43,44] only 5 states and 2 municipalities ever mandated SOGI data be collected at COVID-19 testing or treatment sites,[45] limiting our ability to track these inequities and intervene upon them.[46,47] Even now, as priorities shift to understanding the pandemic's long-term impacts across health, social, and economic domains, the experiences of LGBTQ+ people continue to be erased because of the omission of SOGI measures from population surveys used to monitor such outcomes.[42] Work like the current study can contribute important insights; however, we acknowledge that our data's nonrepresentative nature will fail to make visible the full extent to which the pandemic has harmed structurally marginalized populations. We echo Sell and Krims in naming such gaps as public health malpractice[6] and urge the Centers for Disease Control and Prevention and other institutions to require the collection and reporting of SOGI data in ongoing and future surveillance efforts.

With respect to scholarship, researchers who do have access to pandemic-related SOGI data should analyze them intersectionally (e.g., stratified by multiple dimensions of social position simultaneously and contextualized within systems of power) whenever possible. As we and others have shown,[48] the pandemic's mental health consequences disproportionately burden those marginalized by intersections of heterosexism, sexism, and racism (among other axes of inequity)—ignoring such patterns by assuming within-group homogeneity risks producing ungeneralizable results that could impede actions toward equity. We encourage researchers who are engaged in this work to follow guidelines regarding the incorporation of intersectionality into quantitative study designs and analyses[49–51] and emphasize the importance of clearly articulating potential biases introduced when using nonrepresentative, predominantly White, cisgender, and heterosexual data. We also stress the importance of centering the experiences of impacted communities through equitable partnerships, power sharing, and capacity building.

Finally, it will be essential for public health professionals and communities to collaboratively develop equity-centered mental health interventions as part of ongoing COVID-19 relief efforts and in preparation for future crises. Thus far, interventions aimed at addressing mental health inequities experienced by sexual minorities during the pandemic have focused on bolstering individual-level responses to minority stressors to promote resilience[52,53]; however, informed by intersectional scholarship-activism,[54] we recognize the need to additionally target upstream determinants related to systemic oppression that disproportionately expose structurally marginalized populations to these stressors in the first place.[1] For example, sexual minority women face well-documented barriers to accessing mental health care because of deficits in culturally competent providers and insurance coverage that were further exacerbated by lockdowns and other necessary containment measures[55]; the expansions to telehealth and Medicaid enrollment that occurred in early 2020 were critical to mitigating these inequities and represent key policy levers that can be continued in the postpandemic era.[40] Alongside health care–specific policies, those focused on extending social safety nets (e.g., eviction moratoriums),[38,39] as well as those providing support to community organizations (including LGBTQ+ centers),[56] are known to have positively impacted mental health during the pandemic, and were likely especially salient for sexual minority women of color and other multiply marginalized populations that experienced severe spikes in unemployment, houselessness, food insecurity, and other stressors.[43,44] Future research should be directed toward understanding how this multifaceted pandemic policy environment shaped mental health outcomes for diverse sexual minority people to inform structural interventions that promote intersectional mental health equity, during COVID-19 and beyond. AJPH

ABOUT THE AUTHORS

Ariel L. Beccia is with the Division of Adolescent and Young Adult Medicine, Boston Children's Hospital, Boston, MA. Dougie Zubizarreta is with the Department of Social and Behavioral Sciences, Harvard T. H. Chan School of Public Health, Boston. S. Bryn Austin is with the Division of Adolescent and Young Adult Medicine, Boston Children's Hospital, and Channing Division of Network Medicine, Department of Medicine, Brigham and Women's Hospital and Harvard Medical School, Boston. Julia R. Raifman is with the Department of Health Law, Policy, and Management, Boston University School of Public Health, Boston. Jorge E. Chavarro is with the Department of Nutrition, Harvard T. H. Chan School of Public Health. Brittany M. Charlton is with the Department of Population Medicine, Harvard Medical School and Harvard Pilgrim Health Care Institute, Boston.

CORRESPONDENCE

Correspondence should be sent to Ariel L. Beccia, 1 Autumn St, Boston Children's Hospital, Boston, MA 02215 (e-mail: ariel.beccia@childrens.harvard.edu). Reprints can be ordered at https://ajph.org by clicking the "Reprints" link.

PUBLICATION INFORMATION

Full Citation: Beccia AL, Zubizarreta D, Austin SB, Raifman JR, Chavarro JE, Charlton BM. Trajectories of mental distress among US women by sexual orientation and racialized group during the first year of the COVID-19 pandemic. *Am J Public Health*. 2024;114(5):511–522.

Acceptance Date: January 21, 2024.

DOI: https://doi.org/10.2105/AJPH.2024.307601

CONTRIBUTORS

A. L. Beccia contributed to conceptualization, formal analysis, and visualization and wrote the original draft. A. L. Beccia, D. Zubizarreta, and B. M. Charlton contributed to methodology. S. B. Austin and B. M. Charlton contributed to supervision. All authors reviewed and edited the article.

ACKNOWLEDGMENTS

This work was supported by the National Institute on Minority Health and Health Disparities (1F32MD017452-01, awarded to A. L. Beccia). Other support included grants U01HL145386 and U01CA176726.

The authors would like to acknowledge Janet Rich-Edwards, ScD, MPH, for her leading efforts in launching the COVID-19 Sub-Study and for her feedback on the current study, the members of the Sexual Orientation and Gender Identity and Expression Health Equity Research Collaborative at the Harvard T. H. Chan School for Public Health for their insightful feedback on earlier drafts of this article, and the contributions of the individuals who participated in the COVID-19 Sub-Study.

Note. The content is solely the responsibility of the authors and does not necessarily represent the official views of the National Institutes of Health.

CONFLICTS OF INTEREST

The authors have no potential or actual conflicts of interest to disclose.

HUMAN PARTICIPANT PROTECTION

Protocols for the COVID-19 Sub-Study were approved by the institutional review board of the Brigham and Women's Hospital and Harvard T. H. Chan School of Public Health. Our secondary analyses were exempt from further review. Data access procedures are described at https://nurseshealthstudy.org/researchers.

REFERENCES

1. Phillips G II, Felt D, Ruprecht MM, et al. Addressing the disproportionate impacts of the COVID-19 pandemic on sexual and gender minority populations in the United States: actions toward equity. *LGBT Health*. 2020;7(6):279–282. https://doi.org/10.1089/lgbt.2020.0187
2. Dawson L, Kirzinger A, Kates J. The impact of the COVID-19 pandemic on LGBT people. KFF. 2021. Available at: https://www.kff.org/coronavirus-covid-19/poll-finding/the-impact-of-the-covid-19-pandemic-on-lgbt-people. Accessed August 16, 2023.
3. File T, Marlay M. LGBT adults report anxiety, depression during pandemic. US Census Bureau. 2022. Available at: https://www.census.gov/library/stories/2022/06/lgbt-adults-report-anxiety-depression-during-pandemic.html. Accessed August 16, 2023.
4. Flentje A, Obedin-Maliver J, Lubensky ME, Dastur Z, Neilands T, Lunn MR. Depression and anxiety changes among sexual and gender minority people coinciding with onset of COVID-19 pandemic. *J Gen Intern Med*. 2020;35(9):2788–2790. https://doi.org/10.1007/s11606-020-05970-4
5. Fish JN, Salerno J, Williams ND, et al. Sexual minority disparities in health and well-being as a consequence of the COVID-19 pandemic differ by sexual identity. *LGBT Health*. 2021;8(4):263–272. https://doi.org/10.1089/lgbt.2020.0489
6. Sell RL, Krims EI. Structural transphobia, homophobia, and biphobia in public health practice: the example of COVID-19 surveillance. *Am J Public Health*. 2021;111(9):1620–1626. https://doi.org/10.2105/AJPH.2021.306277
7. Veldhuis CB, Nesoff ED, McKowen ALW, et al. Addressing the critical need for long-term mental health data during the COVID-19 pandemic: changes in mental health from April to September 2020. *Prev Med*. 2021;146:106465. https://doi.org/10.1016/j.ypmed.2021.106465
8. Chang CJ, Feinstein BA, Chu BC, Selby EA. The negative impact of COVID-19 on sexual minority young adults: demographic differences and prospective associations with depression. *Psychol Sex Orientat Gend Divers*. 2021;8(2):220–227. https://doi.org/10.1037/sgd0000494
9. Akré ER, Anderson A, Stojanovski K, Chung KW, VanKim NA, Chae DH. Depression, anxiety, and alcohol use among LGBTQ+ people during the COVID-19 pandemic. *Am J Public Health*. 2021;111(9):1610–1619. https://doi.org/10.2105/AJPH.2021.306394
10. Mooi-Reci I, Risman BJ. The gendered impacts of COVID-19: lessons and reflections. *Gend Soc*. 2021;35(2):161–167. https://doi.org/10.1177/08912432211001305
11. Kamal K, Li JJ, Hahm HC, Liu CH. Psychiatric impacts of the COVID-19 global pandemic on US sexual and gender minority young adults. *Psychiatry Res*. 2021;299:113855. https://doi.org/10.1016/j.psychres.2021.113855
12. Moore SE, Wierenga KL, Prince DM, Gillani B, Mintz LJ. Disproportionate impact of the COVID-19 pandemic on perceived social support, mental health and somatic symptoms in sexual and gender minority populations. *J Homosex*. 2021;68(4):577–591. https://doi.org/10.1080/00918369.2020.1868184
13. Manning WD, Kamp Dush CM. COVID-19 stress and sexual identities. *Socius*. 2022;8. https://doi.org/10.1177/23780231221105376
14. Tai DBG, Sia IG, Doubeni CA, Wieland ML. Disproportionate impact of COVID-19 on racial and ethnic minority groups in the United States: a 2021 update. *J Racial Ethn Health Disparities*. 2022;9(6):2334–2339. https://doi.org/10.1007/s40615-021-01170-w
15. Khazanchi R, Evans CT, Marcelin JR. Racism, not race, drives inequity across the COVID-19 continuum. *JAMA Netw Open*. 2020;3(9):e2019933. https://doi.org/10.1001/jamanetworkopen.2020.19933
16. Thomeer MB, Moody MD, Yahirun J. Racial and ethnic disparities in mental health and mental health care during the COVID-19 pandemic. *J Racial Ethn Health Disparities*. 2023;10(2):961–976. https://doi.org/10.1007/s40615-022-01284-9
17. Nguyen LH, Anyane-Yeboa A, Klaser K, et al. The mental health burden of racial and ethnic minorities during the COVID-19 pandemic. *PLoS One*. 2022;17(8):e0271661. https://doi.org/10.1371/journal.pone.0271661
18. Moreno-Agostino D, Woodhead C, Ploubidis GB, Das-Munshi J. A quantitative approach to the intersectional study of mental health inequalities during the COVID-19 pandemic in UK young adults. *Soc Psychiatry Psychiatr Epidemiol*. 2023; epub ahead of print January 24, 2023. https://doi.org/10.1007/s00127-023-02424-0
19. Brooks V. *Minority Stress and Lesbian Women*. Lexington, MA: Lexington Books; 1981.
20. Rich AJ, Salway T, Scheim A, Poteat T. Sexual minority stress theory: remembering and honoring the work of Virginia Brooks. *LGBT Health*. 2020;7(3):124–127. https://doi.org/10.1089/lgbt.2019.0223
21. Meyer IH. Prejudice, social stress, and mental health in lesbian, gay, and bisexual populations: conceptual issues and research evidence. *Psychol Bull*. 2003;129(5):674–697. https://doi.org/10.1037/0033-2909.129.5.674
22. The Combahee River Collective Statement. 1977. Available at: https://www.loc.gov/item/lcwaN0028151. Accessed August 16, 2023.
23. Collins PH. *Black Feminist Thought: Knowledge, Consciousness, and the Politics of Empowerment*. New York, NY: Routledge; 1990.
24. Crenshaw K. Mapping the margins: intersectionality, identity politics, and violence against women of color. *Stanford Law Rev*. 1991;43(6):1241–1299. https://doi.org/10.2307/1229039
25. Bowleg L. The problem with the phrase women and minorities: intersectionality—an important theoretical framework for public health. *Am J Public Health*. 2012;102(7):1267–1273. https://doi.org/10.2105/AJPH.2012.300750
26. Rich-Edwards JW, Ding M, Rocheleau CM, et al. American frontline healthcare personnel's access to and use of personal protective equipment early in the COVID-19 pandemic. *J Occup Environ Med*. 2021;63(11):913–920. https://doi.org/10.1097/JOM.0000000000002308
27. Bao Y, Bertoia ML, Lenart EB, et al. Origin, methods, and evolution of the three Nurses' Health Studies. *Am J Public Health*. 2016;106(9):1573–1581. https://doi.org/10.2105/AJPH.2016.303338
28. Remafedi G, Resnick M, Blum R, Harris L. Demography of sexual orientation in adolescents. *Pediatrics*. 1992;89(4 pt 2):714–721. https://doi.org/10.1542/peds.89.4.714
29. Kroenke K, Spitzer RL, Williams JBW. The Patient Health Questionnaire-2: validity of a two-item depression screener. *Med Care*. 2003;41(11):1284–1292. https://doi.org/10.1097/01.MLR.0000093487.78664.3C
30. Kroenke K, Spitzer RL, Williams JBW, Monahan PO, Löwe B. Anxiety disorders in primary care: prevalence, impairment, comorbidity, and detection. *Ann Intern Med*. 2007;146(5):317–325. https://doi.org/10.7326/0003-4819-146-5-200703060-00004
31. Yelland LN, Salter AB, Ryan P. Performance of the modified Poisson regression approach for estimating relative risks from clustered prospective data. *Am J Epidemiol*. 2011;174(8):984–992. https://doi.org/10.1093/aje/kwr183
32. Robinson E, Sutin AR, Daly M, Jones A. A systematic review and meta-analysis of longitudinal cohort studies comparing mental health before versus during the COVID-19 pandemic in 2020.

J Affect Disord. 2022;296:567–576. https://doi.org/10.1016/j.jad.2021.09.098

33. Riggle EDB, Drabble LA, Bochicchio LA, et al. Experiences of the COVID-19 pandemic among African American, Latinx, and White sexual minority women: a descriptive phenomenological study. *Psychol Sex Orientat Gend Divers*. 2021;8(2):145–158. https://doi.org/10.1037/sgd0000510
34. Schmitz RM, Gomez G, Propst A, Tabler J, Charak R. Queer politics of a pandemic: LGBTQ+ people's conceptions of COVID-19's politicization. *Sex Res Social Policy*. 2023;20(2):751–765. https://doi.org/10.1007/s13178-022-00719-6
35. Laster Pirtle WN, Wright T. Structural gendered racism revealed in pandemic times: intersectional approaches to understanding race and gender health inequities in COVID-19. *Gend Soc*. 2021;35(2):168–179. https://doi.org/10.1177/08912432211001302
36. Kay JB. "Stay the fuck at home!": feminism, family and the private home in a time of coronavirus. *Fem Media Stud*. 2020;20(6):883–888. https://doi.org/10.1080/14680777.2020.1765293
37. Movement Advancement Project. Under fire: the war on LGBTQ people in America. 2023. Available at: https://www.mapresearch.org/file/Under%20Fire%20report_MAP%202023.pdf. Accessed August 16, 2023.
38. Leifheit KM, Pollack CE, Raifman J, et al. Variation in state-level eviction moratorium protections and mental health among US adults during the COVID-19 pandemic. *JAMA Netw Open*. 2021;4(12):e2139585. https://doi.org/10.1001/jamanetworkopen.2021.39585
39. Donnelly R, Farina MP. How do state policies shape experiences of household income shocks and mental health during the COVID-19 pandemic? *Soc Sci Med*. 2021;269:113557. https://doi.org/10.1016/j.socscimed.2020.113557
40. Goldman ML, Druss BG, Horvitz-Lennon M, et al. Mental health policy in the era of COVID-19. *Psychiatr Serv*. 2020;71(11):1158–1162. https://doi.org/10.1176/appi.ps.202000219
41. Bowleg L, Landers S. The need for COVID-19 LGBTQ-specific data. *Am J Public Health*. 2021;111(9):1604–1605. https://doi.org/10.2105/AJPH.2021.306463
42. Kapadia F. Data democratization for health equity: a public health of consequence, August 2023. *Am J Public Health*. 2023;113(8):839–840. https://doi.org/10.2105/AJPH.2023.307350
43. Movement Advancement Project. The disproportionate impacts of COVID-19 on LGBTQ households in the US 2020. Available at: https://www.lgbtmap.org/2020-covid-lgbtq-households. Accessed August 16, 2023.
44. Sears B, Conron K, Flores A. The impact of the Fall 2020 COVID-19 surge on LGBT adults in the US. The Williams Institute, UCLA. 2021. Available at: https://williamsinstitute.law.ucla.edu/publications/covid-surge-lgbt. Accessed September 1, 2023.
45. Cahill S. Public health is missing crucial data on LGBTQIA+ people. It's not hard to collect. *STAT*. January 14, 2022. Available at: https://www.statnews.com/2022/01/14/public-health-entities-missing-sexual-orientation-gender-identity-data. Accessed August 22, 2023.
46. Cahill SR. Still in the dark regarding the public health impact of COVID-19 on sexual and gender minorities. *Am J Public Health*. 2021;111(9):1606–1609. https://doi.org/10.2105/AJPH.2021.306397
47. Krieger N. ENOUGH: COVID-19, structural racism, police brutality, plutocracy, climate change—and time for health justice, democratic governance, and an equitable, sustainable future. *Am J Public Health*. 2020;110(11):1620–1623. https://doi.org/10.2105/AJPH.2020.305886
48. Parenteau AM, Boyer CJ, Campos LJ, et al. A review of mental health disparities during COVID-19: evidence, mechanisms, and policy recommendations for promoting societal resilience. *Dev Psychopathol*. 2023;35(4):1821–1842. https://doi.org/10.1017/S0954579422000499
49. Bauer GR. Incorporating intersectionality theory into population health research methodology: challenges and the potential to advance health equity. *Soc Sci Med*. 2014;110:10–17. https://doi.org/10.1016/j.socscimed.2014.03.022
50. Agénor M. Future directions for incorporating intersectionality into quantitative population health research. *Am J Public Health*. 2020;110(6):803–806. https://doi.org/10.2105/AJPH.2020.305610
51. Moradi B, Grzanka PR. Using intersectionality responsibly: toward critical epistemology, structural analysis, and social justice activism. *J Couns Psychol*. 2017;64(5):500–513. https://doi.org/10.1037/cou0000203
52. Craig SL, Leung VWY, Pascoe R, et al. AFFIRM Online: utilising an affirmative cognitive–behavioural digital intervention to improve mental health, access, and engagement among LGBTQA+ youth and young adults. *Int J Environ Res Public Health*. 2021;18(4):1541. https://doi.org/10.3390/ijerph18041541
53. Fish JN, King-Marshall EC, Turpin RE, Aparicio EM, Boekeloo BO. Assessing the implementation of an LGBTQ+ mental health services training program to determine feasibility and acceptability during the COVID-19 pandemic [erratum in *Prev Sci*. 2024; epub ahead of print January 8, 2024]. *Prev Sci*. 2023; epub ahead of print March 10, 2023. https://doi.org/10.1007/s11121-023-01505-5
54. Poteat T. Navigating the storm: how to apply intersectionality to public health in times of crisis. *Am J Public Health*. 2021;111(1):91–92. https://doi.org/10.2105/AJPH.2020.305944
55. Ruprecht MM, Wang X, Johnson AK, et al. Evidence of social and structural COVID-19 disparities by sexual orientation, gender identity, and race/ethnicity in an urban environment. *J Urban Health*. 2021;98(1):27–40. https://doi.org/10.1007/s11524-020-00497-9
56. Pachankis JE, Clark KA, Jackson SD, Pereira K, Levine D. Current capacity and future implementation of mental health services in US LGBTQ community centers. *Psychiatr Serv*. 2021;72(6):669–676. https://doi.org/10.1176/appi.ps.202000575

Temporal Trends in Mental Health in the United States by Gender Identity, 2014–2021

Donn Feir, PhD, and Samuel Mann, PhD

Objectives. To examine the temporal trends in the transgender–cisgender mental health disparity in the United States.

Methods. We used 2014–2021 US Behavioral Risk Factor Surveillance System Survey data with logistic and ordinary least squares regression to document temporal trends in the transgender–cisgender disparity in self-reports of the number of poor mental health days in the past month and frequent mental distress.

Results. In 2014, cisgender individuals reported a mean average of 3.68 (95% confidence interval [CI] = 3.65, 3.70) poor mental health days compared with a mean average of 5.42 (95% CI = 4.68, 6.16) poor mental health days among transgender respondents. The size of this disparity adjusted by differences in observable characteristics increased by 2.75 days (95% CI = 0.58, 4.91) over the sample period. In 2014, 11.4% (95% CI = 11.3%, 11.5%) of cisgender adults reported frequent mental distress compared with 18.9% (95% CI = 15.9%, 22%) of transgender adults. By 2021, 14.6% (95% CI = 15.9%, 22%) of cisgender adults and 32.9% (95% CI = 30.7%, 35.1%) of transgender adults reported frequent mental distress.

Conclusions. Policies are needed to address the worsening mental health of transgender and gender-nonconforming people in the United States. (*Am J Public Health*. 2024;114(5):523–526. https://doi.org/10.2105/AJPH.2024.307603)

AJPH May 2024, Vol. 114, No. 5

Gender minority (i.e., transgender, gender diverse, gender-nonconforming and gender nonbinary) adults have higher rates of depression, anxiety, suicidal behavior, substance use, and self-reported poor mental health than do their cisgender counterparts.[1–3] However, most previous work has relied on convenience samples or a single year of data, limiting analysis of temporal trends in transgender mental health disparity. Analysis of temporal trends is needed to inform progress in addressing health disparities among gender minority populations.[4] To our knowledge, this study is the first population-representative analysis of temporal trends in the mental health disparity between cisgender and gender minority populations.

METHODS

In this repeated cross-sectional study, we used yearly probability-based samples from the 2014–2021 Behavioral Risk Factor Surveillance System (BRFSS) from 43 states implementing the optional sexual orientation and gender identity module. The exposure variable was gender minority identity, which was elicited by the question "Do you consider yourself to be transgender?" Outcomes included the number of poor mental health days in the past month (0–30) and frequent mental distress (≥ 14 poor mental health days in the past month).[5] We conducted statistical analysis with Stata version 17.0 (StataCorp LP, College Station, TX). We estimated unadjusted and adjusted models using ordinary least squares for the outcome "number of poor mental health days" and logistic models for the outcome "frequent poor mental health." Negative binomial regression estimated rate ratios for the number of poor mental health days are reported in Appendix Table B (available as a supplement to the online version of this article at http://www.ajph.org). We generated estimates by year, controlling for whether the respondent was contacted via cellphone or landline, state of residence, binary gender (which comes from the question "Are you male or female?"), age (and its quadratic transformation), race and ethnicity, education level, marital status, parenthood, insurance status, income, and state indicators. We generated all estimates using the BRFSS sampling weights.[6]

RESULTS

The sample included 3 402 830 adults of whom 0.24% identified as gender minority. Among the gender minority sample, 3113 identified as transgender men, 3297 identified as transgender women, and 1753 identified as gender nonconforming. Compared with cisgender adults, gender minority adults were more likely to be younger than 24 years and identify as non-White and less likely to have graduated from college, to have a household income greater than $75 000, or to have health insurance (Appendix Table A, available as a supplement to the online version of this article at http://www.ajph.org).

We present the unadjusted and adjusted poor mental health days results in Figure 1, which presents the clear trends visually, showing the growing divide in average mental health measures between gender minority and cisgender respondents. The table portion of Figure 1 presents the underlying means and adjusted and unadjusted changes. In 2014, cisgender individuals reported a mean average of 3.68 (95% confidence interval [CI] = 3.65, 3.70) poor mental health days compared with a mean average of 5.42 (95% CI = 4.48, 6.16) poor mental health days among transgender adults. By 2021, cisgender individuals reported a mean average of 4.61 (95% CI = 4.59, 4.64) poor mental health days compared with a mean average of 9.57 (95% CI = 9.03, 10.11) poor mental health among transgender adults. In fully adjusted models, transgender individuals reported significantly more poor mental health days since 2016. The size of this disparity adjusted by differences in observable characteristics increased by 2.75 days (95% CI = 0.58, 4.91).

Appendix Figure A (available as a supplement to the online version of this article at http://www.ajph.org) demonstrates similar results regarding the proportion reporting frequent mental distress. In 2014, a mean average of 11.4% (95% CI = 11.3%, 11.5%) of cisgender individuals reported frequent mental distress compared with a mean average of 18.9% (95% CI = 15.9%, 22%) of transgender adults. By 2021, a mean average of 14.6% (95% CI = 14.5%, 14.7%) of cisgender individuals reported frequent mental distress compared with a mean average of 32.9% (95% CI = 30.7%, 35.1%) of transgender adults. In fully adjusted models, transgender adults had significantly higher odds of reporting frequent mental distress since 2016.

Appendix Figure B (available as a supplement to the online version of this article at http://www.ajph.org) demonstrates similar patterns for transgender minority, transgender women, and gender-nonconforming populations for the average number of poor mental health days and for the proportion of respondents with frequently poor mental health (Appendix Figure C, available as a supplement to the online version of this article at http://www.ajph.org).

DISCUSSION

We document worsening mental health among gender minority and cisgender populations. These trends are not attributable to changes in the composition of states that ask questions that allow gender minority individuals to be identified. We observed similar trends when we restricted the sample to include only states that asked respondents about gender identity in every year from 2014 to 2021; these trends are presented in Appendix Figure D (available as a supplement to the online version of this article at http://www.ajph.org). Adjusted models also include state indicators.

Findings suggest that disparities in mental health across gender identity have increased over time, despite broad improvements in attitudes toward gender minorities,[7] increasing access to gender-affirming care,[8] and national policy progress.[9] However, the passage of antitransgender legislation over the past 5 years has likely contributed to these worsening trends.[10] During the first 10 months of 2023 alone, there were more than 550 new antitransgender bills introduced,[11] and scholarship indicates negative associations between these bills and mental health outcomes.[10] Although structural factors have likely contributed to the documented disparities, overturning related policies is unlikely to eradicate the disparity. Indeed, even in countries with high levels of protection for transgender individuals (e.g., Denmark), mental health disparities persist.[12] Addressing mental health disparities remains a priority in research and clinical practice, and our findings

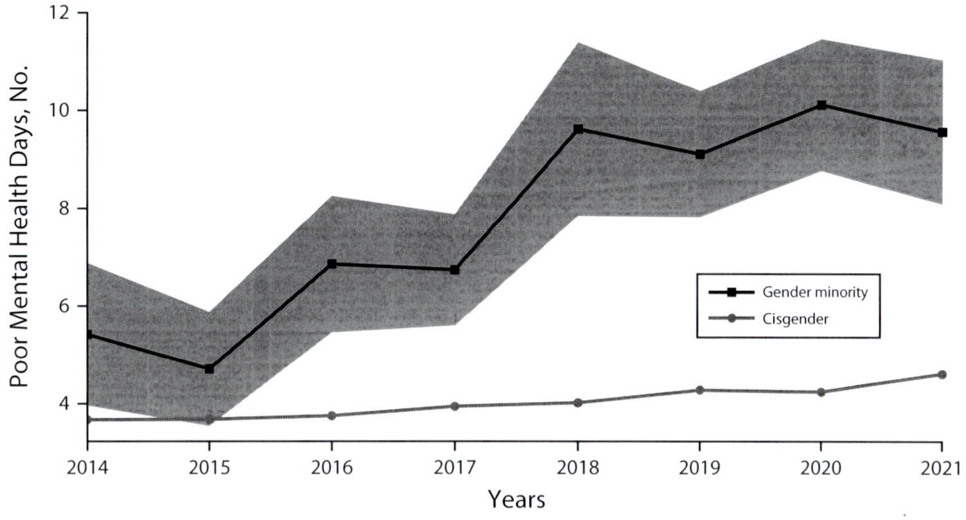

	2014	2015	2016	2017	2018	2019	2020	2021	Change 2014–2021
Cisgender, mean (95% CI)	3.68	3.69	3.76	3.95	4.03	4.28	4.24	4.61	0.94
	(3.65, 3.70)	(3.66, 3.71)	(3.73, 3.78)	(3.92, 3.97)	(4.00, 4.05)	(4.26, 4.31)	(4.22, 4.30)	(4.59, 4.64)	(0.86, 1.02)
Gender minority, mean (95% CI)	5.42	4.71	6.86	6.74	9.62	9.11	10.12	9.57	4.14
	(4.48, 6.16)	(4.07, 5.35)	(6.11, 7.61)	(6.07, 7.41)	(8.90, 10.34)	(8.46, 9.76)	(9.50, 10.74)	(9.03, 10.11)	(2.07, 6.22)
Unadjusted difference (95% CI)	1.75	1.03	3.10	2.80	5.59	4.83	5.87	4.95	3.21
	(0.29, 3.21)	(−0.14, 2.20)	(1.71, 4.50)	(1.66, 3.93)	(3.82, 7.37)	(3.55, 6.12)	(4.52, 7.22)	(3.48, 6.43)	(1.13, 5.28)
Adjusted difference (95% CI)	1.22	0.65	2.35	2.27	4.59	3.77	4.93	3.80	2.75
	(−0.34, 2.77)	(0.53, 1.83)	(0.99, 3.72)	(1.17, 3.38)	(2.91, 6.26)	(2.54, 5.01)	(3.55, 6.30)	(2.41, 5.18)	(0.58, 4.91)
No.	443 601	424 055	466 689	439 543	421 944	401 964	392 360	412 674	856 275

FIGURE 1— Trends Over Time in Mean Average Number of Poor Mental Health Days in the Past 30 Days by Gender Minority Status: United States, BRFSS, 2014–2021

Note. BRFSS = Behavioral Risk Factor Surveillance System; CI = confidence interval. All statistics use BRFSS survey weights. Light gray circles indicate averages for cisgender individuals, and the black squares indicate the means value for all gender minorities. Results for specific groups are reported in the Appendix Figures B and C. The 95% CIs are the shaded reasons around the mean markers and are very narrow for cisgender respondents. Adjusted models for means estimated using ordinary least squares.

demonstrate the need to explore multilevel legal-, clinical-, and community-based approaches to addressing this disparity.

Limitations

This study is subject to several limitations. Our measures of mental health are from self-reports. Future work that can explore whether similar trends are seen using clinical measures would help to further validate our findings. Additionally, we do not have data for 7 states (i.e., Alabama, Maine, Nebraska, New Hampshire, North Dakota, Oregon, and South Dakota) or Washington, DC. This is attributable to states opting to not include the sexual orientation and gender identity module in the BRFSS. Such a decision may be associated with the outcome variables as well as broader stigma toward transgender people. The BRFSS also does not survey people who are unhoused, are incarcerated, or reside in group-living quarters.

Furthermore, although Appendix Figures B and C show that the mental health disparity is most pronounced for gender-nonconforming persons, the limited sample size prevented us from exploring how the documented disparities vary across other demographic groups (e.g., race, sexual orientation). Future work should explore how intersectional identities and associated structural forces affect gender identity–based mental health disparities. Finally, these widening disparities in mental health should be understood in a social context and not used in any fashion that results in increased stigma against the gender minority community.

Public Health Implications

Our findings demonstrate sizable and worsening inequities in mental health across gender identity. Mental health and primary care providers must be prepared to address the unique psychosocial needs of gender minority adults. Furthermore, our findings highlight the need for action to reduce these disparities. Future work that can identify the best approaches to mitigating both external and internal factors that drive mental health disparities for gender minority populations will be critical to developing targeted responses to transgender mental health disparity. AJPH

ABOUT THE AUTHORS

Donn Feir is with the Department of Economics, University of Victoria, Victoria, BC. Samuel Mann is with the RAND Corporation, Arlington, VA.

CORRESPONDENCE

Correspondence should be sent to Samuel Mann, RAND Corporation, 1200 South Hayes St, Arlington, VA 22202 (e-mail: mann@rand.org). Reprints can be ordered at http://www.ajph.org by clicking the "Reprints" link.

PUBLICATION INFORMATION

Full Citation: Feir D, Mann S. Temporal trends in mental health in the United States by gender identity, 2014–2021. *Am J Public Health*. 2024; 114(5):523–526.

Acceptance Date: January 21, 2024.

DOI: https://doi.org/10.2105/AJPH.2024.307603

CONTRIBUTORS

The authors contributed equally to this brief.

ACKNOWLEDGMENTS

The authors would like to thank Aaron Devor and Gilbert Gonzales for helpful comments on a previous draft of this brief.

CONFLICTS OF INTEREST

The authors have no known competing financial interests or personal relationships that could have appeared to influence the work reported in this brief.

HUMAN PARTICIPANT PROTECTION

The study followed the Strengthening the Reporting of Observational Studies in Epidemiology reporting guidelines and did not require ethical approval from an institutional review board because it used de-identified publicly available data.

REFERENCES

1. Proctor K, Haffer SC, Ewald E, Hodge C, James CV. Identifying the transgender population in the Medicare program. *Transgend Health*. 2016;1(1): 250–265. https://doi.org/10.1089/trgh.2016.0031
2. Centers for Disease Control and Prevention. Transgender identity and experiences of violence victimization, substance use, suicide risk, and sexual risk behaviors among high school students—19 states and large urban school districts, 2017. *MMWR Morb Mortal Wkly Rep*. 2019;68(3):67–71. https://doi.org/10.15585/mmwr.mm6803a3
3. Downing JM, Przedworski JM. Health of transgender adults in the U.S., 2014–2016. *Am J Prev Med*. 2018;55(3):336–344. https://doi.org/10.1016/j.amepre.2018.04.045
4. US Institute of Medicine; Committee on Lesbian, Gay, Bisexual, and Transgender Health Issues and Research Gaps and Opportunities. *The Health of Lesbian, Gay, Bisexual, and Transgender People: Building a Foundation for Better Understanding*. Washington, DC: National Academies Press; 2011.
5. Centers for Disease Control and Prevention. Self-reported frequent mental distress among adults-United States, 1993–2001. *MMWR Morb Mortal Wkly Rep*. 2004;53(41):963–966.
6. Centers for Disease Control and Prevention. BRFSS survey data & documentation. Available at: https://www.cdc.gov/brfss/data_documentation/index.htm. Accessed October 19, 2023.
7. Lewis DC, Flores AR, Haider-Markel DP, Miller PR, Taylor JK. Transitioning opinion? *Public Opin Q*. 2022;86(2):343–368. https://doi.org/10.1093/poq/nfac014
8. Canner JK, Harfouch O, Kodadek LM, et al. Temporal trends in gender-affirming surgery among transgender patients in the United States. *JAMA Surg*. 2018;153(7):609–616. https://doi.org/10.1001/jamasurg.2017.6231
9. Cahill S, Miller AS, Keuroghlian AS. Sexual and gender minority health equity in the Biden administration. *JAMA Health Forum*. 2022;3(2): e214868. https://doi.org/10.1001/jamahealthforum.2021.4868
10. Cunningham GB, Watanabe NM, Buzuvis E. Anti-transgender rights legislation and Internet searches pertaining to depression and suicide. *PLoS One*. 2022;17(12):e0279420. https://doi.org/10.1371/journal.pone.0279420
11. Trans Legislation Tracker. 2024 anti-trans bills tracker. Available at: https://translegislation.com. Accessed October 19, 2023.
12. Erlangsen A, Jacobsen AL, Ranning A, Delamare AL, Nordentoft M, Frisch M. Transgender identity and suicide attempts and mortality in Denmark. June 27, 2023. Available at: https://doi.org/10.1001/jama.2023.8627. Accessed February 16, 2024.

State Medicaid Initiatives Targeting Substance Use Disorder in Criminal Legal Settings, 2021

Cashell D. Lewis, MSW, Christina Andrews, PhD, Amanda J. Abraham, PhD, Melissa Westlake, MSW, Faye S. Taxman, PhD, and Colleen M. Grogan, PhD

Objectives. To document state Medicaid pre- and postrelease initiatives for individuals in the criminal legal system with substance use disorder (SUD).

Methods. An Internet-based survey was sent in 2021 to Medicaid directors in all 50 US states and the District of Columbia to determine whether they were pursuing initiatives for persons with SUD across 3 criminal legal settings: jails, prisons, and community corrections. A 90% response rate was obtained.

Results. In 2021, the majority of states did not report any targeted Medicaid initiatives for persons with SUD residing in criminal legal settings. Eighteen states and the District of Columbia adopted at least 1 Medicaid initiative for persons with SUD across the 3 criminal legal settings. The most commonly adopted initiatives were in the areas of medication for opioid use disorder treatment and Medicaid enrollment. Out of 24 possible initiatives for each state (8 initiatives across 3 criminal legal settings), the 2 most commonly adopted were (1) provision of medication treatment of opioid use disorder before release from criminal legal settings (16 states) and (2) facilitation of Medicaid enrollment through suspension rather than termination of Medicaid enrollment upon entry to a criminal legal setting (14 states). Initiatives pertaining to Medicaid SUD care coordination were adopted by the fewest (9) states.

Conclusions. In 2021, states' involvement in Medicaid SUD initiatives for criminal legal populations remained low. Increased adoption of Medicaid SUD initiatives across criminal legal settings is needed, especially knowing the high rate of overdose mortality among this group. (*Am J Public Health.* 2024;114(5):527–530. https://doi.org/10.2105/AJPH.2024.307604)

AJPH May 2024, Vol. 114, No. 5

In 2020, approximately 5.5 million people were incarcerated or serving under community corrections in the United States.[1] Estimates vary, but all studies report an extraordinarily high prevalence of substance use disorder (SUD) among individuals engaged in the criminal legal system. From 2007 to 2009, more than 60% of those residing in prisons and jails had SUD.[2] A 2016 survey of those residing in state and federal prisons similarly reported nearly two thirds (64%) using at least 1 drug in the 30 days before arrest and nearly half (47%) meeting clinical criteria for SUD.[3] The criminal legal–involved populations' risk of overdose is 129 times greater than that of the general population.[4]

As the largest payer of SUD treatment in the United States, Medicaid has played a leading role in expanding access to treatment, particularly in states that have expanded Medicaid.[5] However, the Medicaid Inmate Exclusion Act of 1965, which disallows Medicaid coverage for incarcerated populations, has resulted in approximately 80% of those released from criminal legal settings reentering the community without health insurance.[6] Because individuals face a number of barriers to enrolling and receiving Medicaid-covered services,[7] evidence suggests that securing Medicaid coverage before release can improve treatment access for individuals reentering the community after incarceration.[8,] Among incarcerated adults with a history of SUD, the likelihood of visiting an SUD treatment outpatient facility within the first 30 days of release increased by approximately 8%

after implementation of prerelease Medicaid enrollment assistance.[8]

Although many states have submitted proposals to waive the Medicaid inmate exclusion provision (4 approved in 2023 and 14 pending),[9] states continue to have the option to adopt a number of prerelease and reentry Medicaid initiatives focused on individuals with SUD using sources other than federal Medicaid funds.[10] However, to our knowledge, no previous data are available describing what initiatives states have adopted to enroll and connect criminal legal system populations to Medicaid SUD services or how implementation varies across criminal legal settings (e.g., prisons, jails, and community corrections).

METHODS

Our research team conducted an Internet-based survey of Medicaid programs in the 50 states and the District of Columbia. Each state Medicaid director was emailed a packet that contained a study description, an invitation to participate, and a request to send the survey link to the most knowledgeable staff person or persons. Follow-up emails and phone calls were made to fill in missing data. Forty-six Medicaid programs responded for a survey response rate of 90%.

The survey asked if the state Medicaid program was involved in any SUD initiatives for criminal legal–involved populations. If the state answered "yes," we inquired about 8 initiatives. If the state selected "no" or left the answer blank, we counted the state as not being involved in any initiatives. The initiatives fell into 3 main categories. First, respondents were asked about medication for opioid use disorder (MOUD) treatment—specifically, whether they

1. provide MOUD before release for individuals leaving criminal legal system settings and
2. provide MOUD for individuals residing in criminal legal settings.

Second, we asked about Medicaid enrollment, including whether states

3. suspend or reclassify Medicaid enrollees upon entry to enable coverage,
4. enroll persons before release, and
5. assign Medicaid application counselors.

Third, we asked respondents about SUD care coordination initiatives, including whether they

6. provide SUD care coordination planning as part of discharge planning,
7. assign individuals to Medicaid Health Homes with emphasis on SUD treatment, and
8. assign individuals to a Medicaid managed care plan.

For each initiative, we asked about adoption across 3 settings: jails (preconviction and short-term sentences), prisons (settings for individuals convicted of a felony), and community corrections (resident population under correctional supervision)[11] (for exact wording of survey questions, see the Supplemental Instrument, available as a supplement to the online version of this article at https://ajph.org).

RESULTS

Eighteen states (AZ, CA, IL, LA, MA, MD, MO, MT, ND, NJ, NM, NV, NY, OH, RI, UT, VA, and VT) and the District of Columbia adopted at least 1 Medicaid initiative for criminal legal–involved populations. The most commonly adopted initiatives (17 states) were in the areas of MOUD treatment and Medicaid enrollment (Table 1).

Out of 24 possible initiatives for each state (8 initiatives across 3 criminal legal settings), states most commonly supported the following initiatives: (1) provision of MOUD just before release (16 states in at least 1 setting) or during residence in criminal legal settings (14 states in at least 1 setting), and (2) facilitation of Medicaid enrollment through suspension rather than termination of Medicaid enrollment upon entry to a criminal legal setting (14 states in at least 1 setting) or providing prerelease enrollment into Medicaid (13 states in at least 1 setting).

Eleven states adopted at least 1 SUD care coordination initiative with discharge SUD planning being the most common (9 states in at least 1 setting). Initiatives were most commonly adopted in prison settings, followed by jails, and then community corrections.

DISCUSSION

Given the high rates of overdose mortality among this population, there is an urgent need to provide SUD treatment before release and a clear SUD care coordination plan upon release. Despite this urgent need, the majority of states have no Medicaid initiatives targeted for persons with SUD in criminal legal settings. Among the 19 states that have adopted Medicaid initiatives, they most commonly focus on prison settings, followed by jails. There is 1 exception to this pattern: suspending and reclassifying as opposed to terminating Medicaid enrollment upon entry was more commonly adopted in jails, which makes sense considering jail sentences can be as short as 1 day. The higher involvement in prisons and jails is to be

TABLE 1— Number of US States Adopting Specific Medicaid-Covered Criminal Legal Initiative for Persons With Substance Use Disorder (SUD) as of 2021

Type of Initiative	Total No. of States Adopting in at Least 1 Setting	Total No. of States Adopting in Prisons	Total No. of States Adopting in Jails	Total No. of States Adopting in Community Corrections
Any of the 2 initiatives related to MOUD treatment	17	14	14	9
MOUD prerelease treatment	16	14	12	8
MOUD treatment residing in these settings	14	12	10	7
Any of the 3 initiatives related to Medicaid enrollment	17	16	15	11
Suspend or reclassify	14	12	13	8
Prerelease enrollment	13	12	10	5
Onsite application counselor	8	7	6	4
Any of the 3 initiatives related to SUD care coordination	11	10	8	4
Discharge SUD planning	9	8	5	4
Assign to MCO	6	6	5	1
Assign to SUD health home	2	2	2	2

Note. MCO = managed care organization; MOUD = medication for opioid use disorder.

expected given restrictions from the Inmate Exclusion Act and findings reporting extremely high incidence of overdose rates upon release from these settings. Nonetheless, although the lower adoption of initiatives embedded in community corrections may logically reflect a less urgent need compared with initiatives in jails and prisons, it may also reflect a lost opportunity to improve continuity of Medicaid coverage and service provision, especially since this population is often highly mobile and, thus, difficult to reach once in the community corrections setting.

Only a handful of states adopted SUD care coordination models for criminal legal-involved populations. This may improve over time as Medicaid initiatives may choose to focus first on getting criminal legal–involved populations enrolled and on MOUD and then, as a second step, engaged with care coordination models. Future research should study Medicaid initiatives that provide care coordination in addition to enrollment and MOUD to determine if this comprehensive approach is more effective in reducing overdose rates and moving persons toward recovery.

Finally, all states (and DC) with SUD Medicaid initiatives for criminal legal-involved populations are Medicaid expansion states. While noteworthy, this relationship is expected because single adults are not eligible for Medicaid in nonexpansion states.

PUBLIC HEALTH IMPLICATIONS

Medicaid coverage for criminal legal–involved populations before release (just 1 of the 8 initiatives reported here) is associated with higher health service usage among the population.[8] Coordination between these 2 disparate systems also increases the possibility for continuity of care, and there is some evidence that Medicaid coverage reduces recidivism.[12] Given these public health benefits, lack of state adoption of Medicaid initiatives across criminal legal settings is concerning, and further study of state initiatives targeting this population is crucial. AJPH

ABOUT THE AUTHORS

Cashell D. Lewis is with Crown Family School of Social Work, Policy, and Practice, University of Chicago, IL. Christina Andrews and Melissa Westlake are with the Department of Health Services Policy and Management at Arnold School of Public Health, University of South Carolina, Columbia. Amanda J. Abraham is with the Department of Public Administration and Policy in the School of Public and International Affairs, University of Georgia, Athens. Faye S. Taxman is with the Schar School of Policy and Government and Center for Advancing Correctional Excellence!, George Mason University, Fairfax, VA. Colleen M. Grogan is with Crown Family School of Social Work, Policy, and Practice and the Center for Health Administration Studies, University of Chicago.

CORRESPONDENCE

Correspondence should be sent to Cashell D. Lewis, Crown Family School of Social Work, Policy & Practice, University of Chicago, 969 E 60th St, Chicago, IL 60637 (e-mail: cashell@uchicago.edu). Reprints can be ordered at https://ajph.org by clicking the "Reprints" link.

PUBLICATION INFORMATION

Full Citation: Lewis CD, Andrews C, Abraham AJ, Westlake M, Taxman FS, Grogan CM. State Medicaid initiatives targeting substance use disorder in criminal legal settings, 2021. *Am J Public Health*. 2024;114(5):527–530.

Acceptance Date: January 21, 2024.

DOI: https://doi.org/10.2105/AJPH.2024.307604

CONTRIBUTORS

C. D. Lewis and C. M. Grogan contributed to the study conceptualization and design. C. Andrews, A. J. Abraham, M. Westlake, F. S. Taxman, and C. M. Grogan contributed to data collection. C. D. Lewis, C. M. Grogan, C. Andrews, and A. J. Abraham contributed to analysis and interpretation of results. C. D. Lewis prepared the draft article. All authors reviewed the results and approved the final version of the article.

ACKNOWLEDGMENTS

This study was funded under the Justice Community Opioid Innovation Network (JCOIN) cooperative agreement, funded at the National Institute on Drug Abuse (NIDA) by the National Institutes of Health (NIH). The authors gratefully acknowledge the collaborative contributions of NIDA and support from the following grant awards (U2CDA050097, MPI: Taxman and Rudes; U2CDA050097, MPI: Schneider and Pollack). This grant, NIH NIDA JCOIN 025: R01 DA034634-01, "Mapping Federal Opioid Investments" (PI: Grogan), is a supplement to the Coordination and Translation Center from the Bureau of Justice Assistance to the NIDA JCOIN.

Note. The contents of this publication are solely the responsibility of the authors and do not necessarily represent the official views of NIDA, NIH, or the participating sites.

CONFLICTS OF INTEREST

The authors report no conflicts of interest.

HUMAN PARTICIPANT PROTECTION

No human participants were used in this study.

REFERENCES

1. Kluckow R, Zeng Z. Correctional populations in the United States, 2020. Washington, DC; Bureau of Justice Statistics, US Department of Justice; 2022.
2. Bronson J, Stroop J, Zimmer S, Berzofsky M. Drug use, dependence, and abuse among state prisoners and jail inmates, 2007–2009: special report. Washington, DC: Bureau of Justice Statistics, US Department of Justice; 2017.
3. Maruschak LM, Bronson J, Alper M. Alcohol and drug use and treatment reported by prisoners: survey of prison inmates, 2016. Washington, DC: Bureau of Justice Statistics, US Department of Justice; July 2021.
4. Binswanger IA, Stern MF, Deyo RA, et al. Release from prison—a high risk of death for former inmates. *N Engl J Med*. 2007;356(2):157–165. https://doi.org/10.1056/NEJMsa064115
5. Ortega A. Medicaid expansion and mental health treatment: evidence from the Affordable Care Act. *Health Econ*. 2023;32(4):755–806. https://doi.org/10.1002/hec.4633
6. Albertson EM, Scannell C, Ashtari N, Barnert E. Eliminating gaps in Medicaid coverage during reentry after incarceration. *Am J Public Health*. 2020;110(3):317–321. https://doi.org/10.2105/AJPH.2019.305400
7. Wakeman SE, McKinney ME, Rich JD. Filling the gap: the importance of Medicaid continuity for former inmates. *J Gen Intern Med*. 2009;24(7):860–862. https://doi.org/10.1007/s11606-009-0977-x
8. Burns ME, Cook S, Brown LM, et al. Association between assistance with Medicaid enrollment and use of health care after incarceration among adults with a history of substance use. *JAMA Netw Open*. 2022;5(1):e2142688. https://doi.org/10.1001/jamanetworkopen.2021.42688
9. Kaiser Family Foundation. Medicaid waiver tracker: approved and pending section 1115 waivers by state. 2023. Available at: https://www.kff.org/medicaid/issue-brief/medicaid-waiver-tracker-approved-and-pending-section-1115-waivers-by-state Accessed November 12, 2023.
10. US Department of Health and Human Services, Office of the Assistant Secretary for Planning and Evaluation. Health care transitions for individuals returning to the community from a public institution: promising practices identified by the Medicaid Reentry Stakeholder Group. 2023. Available at: https://aspe.hhs.gov/sites/default/files/documents/d48e8a9fdd499029542f0a30aa78bfd1/health-care-reentry-transitions.pdf. Accessed January 7, 2024.
11. Kaeble D. Probation and parole in the United States, 2021. Bureau of Justice Statistics. 2023. Available at: https://bjs.ojp.gov/library/publications/probation-and-parole-united-states-2021. Accessed April 2, 2023.
12. Aslim EG, Mungan MC, Navarro CI, Yu H. The effect of public health insurance on criminal recidivism. *J Policy Anal Manage*. 2022;41(1):45–91. https://doi.org/10.1002/pam.22345

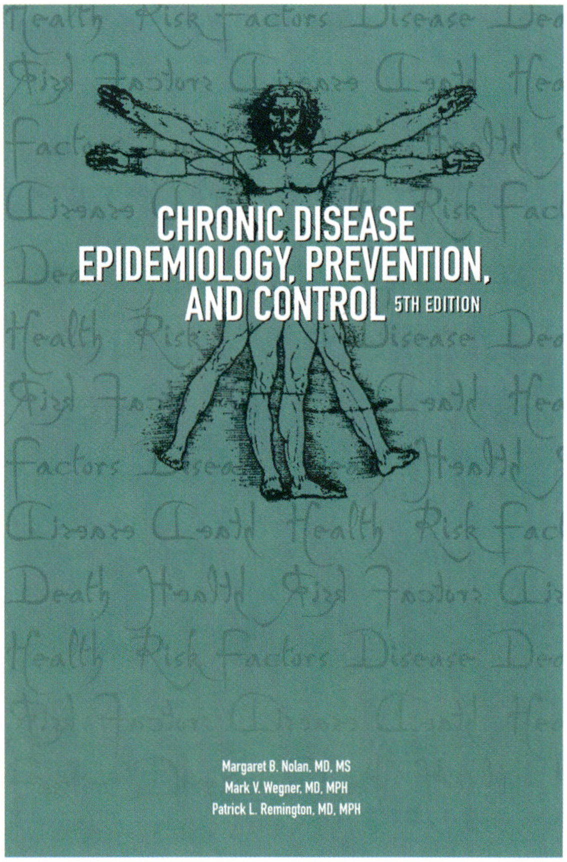

2023, SOFTCOVER, 978-087553-3360

Chronic Disease Epidemiology, Prevention, and Control, 5th edition

Edited by Margaret B. Nolan, MD, MS, Mark V. Wegner, MD, MPH, and Patrick L. Remington, MD, MPH

The fifth edition of *Chronic Disease Epidemiology, Prevention, and Control* has been updated. Its original content has been expanded to include new chapters on often overlooked chronic disease topics such as sleep and oral health. With an enhanced focus on health equity and social determinants of health, as well as the impact of the COVID-19 pandemic on chronic disease prevention and control, this manual is bound to serve as an effective guide for public health practitioners.

APHABOOKSTORE.ORG

APHA PRESS

AN IMPRINT OF **AMERICAN PUBLIC HEALTH ASSOCIATION**